SECRETS
OF THE
CHINESE HERBALISTS

SECRETS OF THE CHINESE HERBALISTS

Richard Lucas

Plant Drawings by Steven Talbott

Parker Publishing Company, Inc.

West Nyack, New York

Library of Congress Cataloging in Publication Data

Lucas, Richard Melvin
   Secrets of the Chinese herbalists.

   Includes index.
   1. Herbs--Therapeutic use. 2. Materia medica,
Vegetable--China. 3. Botany, Medical--China. I. Ti-
tle.
RM666.H33L8   615'.321'0951   76-25955
ISBN 0-13-797639-9

INTRODUCTION

Sir Winston Churchill once observed that, "The farther you look back, the farther forward you can see."

In the past few years there has been a marked interest in the traditional medicines of China, a trend which seems to be accelerating. The first of the ancient Chinese healing arts to capture the attention of Western physicians was acupuncture, and, in the opinion of Dr. E. Grey Dimond, the next will be Chinese herb remedies.

A study of the history of Western orthodox medical science shows that many treatments once considered to be nothing more than superstitious nonsense were later "rediscovered" to become pillars of acceptable health care. With illness and disease so widespread today, it is my contention that the relief of human suffering should be the direct concern of science and less emphasis should be placed on whether the remedy is orthodox or unorthodox. For what does it matter, so long as the treatment is safe and helpful? That is why I have undertaken this monumental task of research and reporting, collecting a mass of information on Oriental herb remedies, and why I wish to share this knowledge with you.

The preparation of this book covered a period of several years. To give you some idea of what was involved, my research included the tedious job of digging through volumes of Oriental herb writings and related sources from the earliest times to the most up-to-date, carefully sorting, cross-checking, translating, and recording pertinent information on the background, history, and value of the Chinese herbal *materia medica*. It was also essential to seek out, in the Chinese sections of certain cities, medical herbalists who could provide me with more direct information. Repeated, lengthy, in-depth consultations with these Chinese practitioners proved highly rewarding. Herb formulas which could be used as domestic self-help remedies, plus fascinating suggestions for healthful, natural living were revealed to me.

Along with many other things, there was the task of gathering together numerous reports on the scientific studies of a variety of Chinese herbs, in which some plants were demonstrated to be medically effective, while others were still to be evaluated. These documents were obtained from accredited sources in many parts of the world.

In the end, the over-all picture became apparent: The Chinese herbalist provides a system of health care that is natural, sensible, and beneficial.

Now, here in this illustrated book, you have at your fingertips a compendium of Chinese herb remedies for coping with a wide variety of health problems. (No attempt has been made to include complex formulas or highly potent single herbs which should be used only under the personal supervision of a Chinese herbalist.)

Many impressive case histories are also presented, in which people in poor health who did not respond to orthodox medicine obtained good results from the use of a natural Chinese herb remedy.

Along with ample coverage of herb recipes that can easily be prepared right in your own home, this book contains information on certain Oriental herb products which are sold on the market in the form of fluid extracts, compounds, blends, syrups, ointments, and so forth. In addition, there is a chapter on herbal tonics which are readily available, to help give you the energy and go-power that will add zest and sparkle to your daily living.

Constipation is, perhaps, the most common health problem in our country. In a great many cases, this condition has been overcome by the correct intake of natural foods and/or specific Chinese herb remedies which are cited in Chapter 11.

Another chapter provides you with a treasure trove of information on an herb prized for thousands of years in the Orient as a longevity plant, a sex rejuvenant, and a preventative as well as a corrective of numerous ailments. Here you'll also learn that certain modern scientific studies have confirmed many of the Chinese claims for the therapeutic power of this remarkable herb.

It is well known that many orthodox tranquilizers and similar drugs prescribed by Western medics for conditions commonly called "nerves" produce dangerous side effects or are habit forming. However, in this book you'll discover that there are Chinese herb remedies which can be used with safety to treat such conditions as stress, nervous headache, insomnia, nervous irritability, and so on.

In addition, there is a chapter devoted specifically to health suggestions and the usage of Chinese herbs for female ailments, and another specialized chapter covering disorders of the male.

All this and much, much more is contained between the covers of this book.

Granted not everything will work for everyone (there are too many individual differences, too many variables), so you will notice the majority of chapters include listings of several different herb remedies for each particular ailment cited. In this way, a person may select one of the remedies or herbal products most appropriate for his or her own individual need, and if after giving it a sufficient trial it does not help, a switch can be made to another. This procedure does not, of course, guarantee success, but it does increase an individual's chances of finding a remedy that might prove helpful.

In case you are wondering whether it will be difficult to locate the various herbs and herbal products mentioned in the following pages, the answer is no. Health food stores carry many of these items, and for your further convenience a list of herb dealers is given at the back of this book.

In closing, I wish to stress what I have said in my previous health books: I do not prescribe. As an author and reporter, I simply pass on to you the findings and experiences of others who have achieved various degrees of success with the use of natural Chinese remedies.

Richard Lucas

TABLE OF CONTENTS

SECRETS
OF THE
CHINESE HERBALISTS

1

THE WISDOM
OF CHINESE HERBALISTS

Some years ago William Engle, the science editor of *American Weekly*, related the following story in that magazine:

Little Pao Ping lay dying of a deadly brain infection. Her doctors, modern men of science at Children's Hospital in Peking, had exhausted all their resources . . .

A call went out to a specialist in herbs and roots, buds, leaves and berries, a healer known as Dr. Chiang Chien-an.

"The child has encephalitis-B," Dr. Pei Li, head of the hospital's encephalitis-B ward, told the herbalist. "We think she can live no more than a day or two."

Dr. Chiang examined the little girl gravely.

"I can cure," he said. "I shall give white tiger soup."

He mixed the ingredients of this potion and of others. He put in gypsum, rice powder, dried gold-and-silver blossoms, wild *shou tan* buds and mulberry leaves to lower temperature; roots of the wild herbs, *yuan sheng* and *sheng ti,* to give energy; camphor from Borneo to calm nerves; ginseng roots to build resistance; and *pei lan,* a fragrant orchid, to combat infection.

Nine days later, Pao Ping was discharged as well.

Mere chance? A one-in-a-million bit of luck? Well, according to an official medical association report, 32 other boys and girls in the same hospital, between the ages of 1 and 14, were also saved from an encephalitis death in this seemingly primitive and fantastic way.[1]

---

[1]Engle, William, Science Editor, "The Search for Life-giving Herbs," *The American Weekly,* November 15, 1959.

Other Impressive Reports

• In the ancient text, the *Pen Ts'ao Ching,* Emperor Shen-ung prescribed the herb Chang Shan (a species of hydrangea) for malaria. Modern scientific research tested this plant and found that the root contained anti-malarial properties.

• Sixteen cases of bacillary dysentary were treated with an ancient Chinese herb mixture which included white peony root, coptis teeta root, and other ingredients. The patients' temperatures became normal within 36 hours, and bowel activity was restored to normal in about four and a half days.

• The preparation of a powder from magaimo (Chinese yam) was found to be effective in treating ulcers. Five patients with duodenal ulcers and fifteen patients with gastric ulcers were treated with two grams of yam powder five times a day for three days. Symptoms were relieved within one week, and X-ray examination showed complete or partial healing of ulcers in four or five weeks.

• In Tientsin, 300 cases of appendicitis were treated with a Chinese herb decoction. The number of leucocytes decreased, temperature was lower, pain vanished, and urination increased. Scientific analyses of the Chinese herb remedy showed that its power in checking the growth of bacteria was greater than that of penicillin.

Widespread Interest in Chinese Herb Medicine

Countless reports such as those cited have produced a continuing and widespread scientific interest in the Chinese materia medica. Dr. Anne A. Cummings, member of a British medical research team sent to Red China, was deeply impressed with her observations of Chinese medicines derived from herbs, roots, and barks. "The Chinese," she said, "have great respect for what they call the 'wisdom of the ancients.'" She explained that they study ancient theories with great interest and try to develop modern techniques for applying them. "The results are nothing short of miraculous," she added.

After returning from a visit to China, Dr. E. Grey Dimond, American heart specialist, had this to say: "Most of the people in that huge country still get most of their medicinal care from doctors who go into the hills and make their own medicines from substances they've been using for 2,000 years. I thought to myself, 'By God, we in the West had to learn to use primitive herbs in digitalis, in ephedrine, and the rauwolfia tranquilizers; there must be a lot of pharmacology the Chinese can teach us too.' " Dr. Dimond reported that he was greatly impressed with a Chinese herb remedy used for the treatment of heart ailments.

The Soviet Academy of Science is also keenly interested in the traditional Chinese materia medica and is deeply engaged in researching this ancient healing art. I.I. Fedorov stated that, "Chinese medicine is the result of countless centuries of valuable practical experience, and once properly evaluated by modern research, it could enrich medical knowledge the world over."

Interest in the Chinese materia medica is also rapidly growing in France, Germany, and other European nations.

THE WISDOM OF THE ANCIENTS

The practice of herbal medicine dates back to the very earliest periods of Chinese history, and over a great span of time many pharmacopoeias were written and revised. Of these works, the oldest is the *Pen Ts'ao Ching,* in which the Red Emperor, Shen-ung, described various medicaments and included instructions for their use. Shen-ung died in the year 2697 B.C. and was succeeded by Huang Ti, the Yellow Emperor, who reigned from about 2697 to 2595 B.C. He composed the celebrated *Nei Ching (The Yellow Emperor's Book of Internal Medicine).* This was later divided into two main sections referred to as *Su Wen* and *Ling Shu.*

A striking similarity with modern thought on preventive medicine can be found in the remarkable *Nei Ching* manual. It states that the human body can be protected against disease by adaption to environmental changes. Ailments must be cured before they arise, says the *Nei Ching,* by proper diet, rest, and work, and by keeping the mind and heart calm. To cure an illness after it arises is like forging weapons after the battle has started or digging a well after you have become thirsty.

And in the *Su Wen,* the first part of the *Nei Ching,* we find the following question asked by Emperor Huang Ti: "I have heard that in ancient times human beings lived to the age of a hundred. In our time we are exhausted at the age of fifty. Is this because of changes in circumstances, or is it the fault of man?" His physician, Ch'i Po, answered: "In ancient times, men lived in accordance with the Tao, the 'Principle.' They observed the law of Yang and Yin, were sober, and led regular, simple lives. For that reason, being healthy in body and mind, they could live to the age of a hundred. In our time, men drink alcohol as if it were water, seek all pleasures, and abandon themselves to intemperance. The sages teach that one must lead a simple and peaceful life. Thus keeping all its energy in reserve, the body cannot be attacked by illness . . . By living in such simplicity, men can still reach the age of a hundred in our time."

Modern Medical Discoveries Known to Ancients

The *Nei Ching* described the circulation of the blood through the body, which was not discovered by the Western world (by Harvey) until the sixteenth century A.D.

Anesthetics were administered by Chinese surgeons as far back as the third century B.C., and the catheter, which the West invented in 1885, was described in *The Thousand Golden Remedies* in the seventh century B.C.

Another remarkable fact is that the concept of psychosomatic ailments (stress-induced illnesses), generally believed to be a modern medical discovery, was known to Chinese healers thousands of years ago. This can be seen very clearly in the following passage from the *Su Wen:* "We must know how to determine whether a disorder is caused by perverse energy coming from the outside [e.g., wind, cold, dampness, heat, dryness], or by emotional stress. Psychic disturbances, like perverse energies, can give rise to muscular disorders and all sorts of illness."

Diagnosis by Pulse

The taking of the pulse was discovered by Pien Ch'ueh, a famous physician of the second century A.D. According to ancient Chinese chronicles, Pien Ch'ueh saved the life of a prince who was unconscious and given up for dead by his court physician. Pien Ch'ueh felt the pulse, found that the prince was still alive, and administered treatment which brought about his recovery.

In the centuries that followed, the method of taking the pulse was highly developed into an intricate system of diagnosis. This system is still practiced today by Chinese healers. With his right hand the herbalist feels the patient's left pulse, and with his left hand he feels the right pulse. He places three fingers—the index, middle, and ring finger—over the pulse and applies weak, moderate, and strong pressure with each finger. The position of the finger and the amount

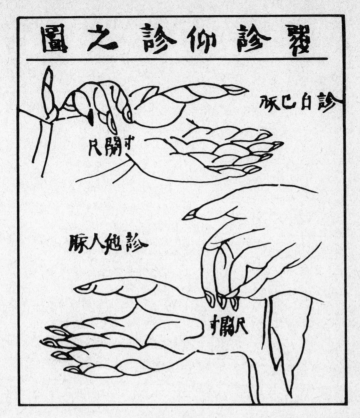

圖之診仰診覆

脉已白診

尺關寸

脉人觑診

寸關尺

Taking the Pulse

of pressure applied reveal the condition of various parts of the body, such as the stomach, spleen, gall bladder, liver, large intestine, small intestine, heart, and so on.

The Pen Ts'ao Kang Mu

As time passed, Chinese healers, each in their own generation, collected the medicinal knowledge of earlier periods and supplemented it with their own findings. In this way, the number of Chinese pharmacopoeias continued to increase and expand. Although each was important, the most outstanding of all is the immense work titled the *Pen Ts'ao Kang Mu* or *General Compendium of Remedies,* published in China in the sixteenth century A.D. It is composed of 56 chapters containing 1,100 illustrations and nearly 12,000 formulas, the result of more than twenty-five years of labor by Li Shih Ch'en, a physician and pharmacologist who catalogued the remedies

of previous eras together with his own discoveries. When treating
patients, Li Shih Chen often preferred to be paid for his services by
obtaining information of any remedies the patient might have heard
of. He then carefully wrote down the recipe and later tested and
evaluated it.

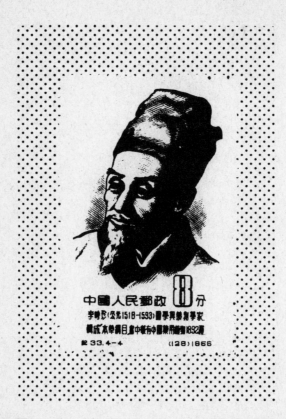

Enlarged Reproduction of Postage Stamp Honoring Li Shih Chen

Today the pharmacopoeia of Li Shih Chen is still considered
highly important to the Chinese materia medica. Modern Western
science has established that many of the herbs listed in the *Pen Ts'ao
Kang Mu* contain valuable medicinal properties. In 1956, the People's
Republic of China honored Li Shih Chen by issuing a postage stamp
bearing his image.

The Chinese Concept of Yang-Yin

Five thousand years experience of compounding and processing roots and herbs has taught the Chinese many things about the rhythm and balance of nature. According to Oriental philosophy, there are two basic and opposing principles that regulate the Universe, and all phenomena are created by their continuous interplay. These two principles, called Yang and Yin, are natural opposites and may be briefly defined as follows (a complete list of Yang-Yin contraries would be endless).

> YANG—Male, light, hot, strong, positive, active, sun, spring, summer.
>
> YIN—Female, dark, cold, weak, negative, passive, earth, autumn, winter.

The Chinese texts explain, "If Yin and Yang are not in harmony, it is as though there were no autumn opposite the spring, no winter opposite the summer." Although Yang and Yin may be opposites, they are not hostile to one another..Each needs the other; without one, the other could not exist. Yang is not superior to Yin, nor is Yin superior to Yang.

Man is a miniature Universe, a microcosm or "small world" in relation to the "greater world" or macrocosm. Being an integral part of the whole, he is subject to the same Cosmic laws. As the whole order of the Universe results from the perfect balance between the two forces of Yin-Yang, so the health of man depends on the equilibrium of Yin-Yang in his body.

Incorrect Balance between Yin and Yang
Results in Illness

The Chinese believe that the action of these dual forces on the human level manifests through the various organs of the body, such as the heart, lungs, spleen, kidneys, stomach, and so on. For example, the contraction (systol) and dilation (diastol) of the heart, which follow each other rhythmically to circulate the blood; the rhythm of inhalation and exhalation of the lungs; the functions of the sympathetic and parasympathetic nervous systems; the act of waking and sleeping.

According to the Chinese, all diseases are the result of a disturbed harmony between Yin and Yang in the body. For example, if the Yin principle in the body predominates, there is weakness, exhaustion, debility; if the Yang predominates, there is irritability and excitation. The ancient medical book, the *Nei Ching,* states: "If Yang is predominant, then the body will grow hot, the pores close and the patient begins to breathe heavily and gasp for breath. Fever will arise, the palate will become dry; the person becomes tense and irritable."

Comparison with Modern Scientific Concepts

This Chinese concept that disease will result if the Yin-Yang balance in the body is disturbed is remarkable when you consider that modern 20th century science is saying practically the same thing. When science discovered the important functions of the sympathetic and parasympathetic nervous systems, the relation to the Chinese theory of Yin-Yang became quite striking. Many physicians are convinced that if the sympathetic and parasympathetic nervous systems are not in harmony with each other, illness will surely follow. Stress diseases which are so rampant today—high blood pressure, heart trouble, stomach ulcers, headaches, insomnia, and so forth—are believed to be partly due to an impaired nervous system caused by the stress and tension of modern living. Science tells us that a harmonious functioning of the nervous systems and a well-balanced disposition are essential to good health.

Yang-Yin Symbol

The Yang-Yin symbol is generally depicted by a circle divided into two parts, one black and the other white, each of which resembles a comma or a fish. The circle represents the Universe (without beginning or end), and the dark and light divisions within it represent the Yang-Yin.

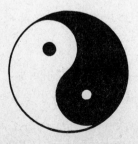

Basic Yin-Yang Symbol

Another Yang-Yin symbol is called the pentagram. It was devised by a Chinese emperor around the year 2900 B.C. It consists of combinations of broken lines (Yin) and straight lines (Yang) surrounding a circle and its two divisions, making a perfect emblem of the balancing of the forces of the Universe.

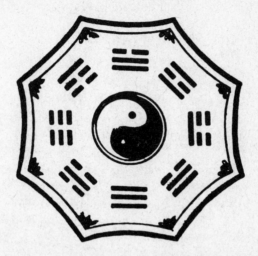

Pentagram—Another Type of Yin-Yang Symbol

In China, the dressing used for the treatment of a fracture or wound often bears a Yang-Yin symbol.

Yang-Yin Guidelines

The concept of Yang-Yin has guided everything Chinese, from government to family relations, from music to art, farming, health, and healing. This is the philosophy which Chinese housewives use to balance their families' diets for health. Many of the roots and herbs they use in supplementing and flavoring the daily meals are the very same as those used by herbalists when preparing herb teas or herbal blends, and the same careful attention to balance is followed by both.

As a result of their age-old Yang-Yin theory, Chinese herbalists do not claim to cure anything. They simply work to support and assist Nature in her endeavor to heal the ailing organism. Since natural foods—e.g., vegetables, fruits, legumes, and herbs—are live substances which have been formulated by countless ages of evolution, the herbalists of China believe that non-poisonous plant medicines supply to the body the appropriate constituents it lacks, in a way similar to that of natural foods. Thus, by providing the body with what it needs or what it cannot produce in sufficient quantities, the Yang-Yin vital force is harmonized, strengthened, and sustained in an indirect way. This method embraces prevention as well as healing. The great modern Chinese scholar, Lin Yutang, wrote: "The Chinese do not draw any distinction between food and medicine. What is good for the body is medicine and at the same time food."

Basic Rules for Preparing Chinese Herb Teas

Generally, Chinese remedies consist of one principal herb or root and at least three or more assistant herbs, roots, or other natural substances. However, there are instances where less are used, and in some cases a domestic remedy may consist of one single botanical (ginseng root and garlic are among a number of such examples).

In preparing the herb teas, aluminum utensils are never used. The most satisfactory, according to the Chinese, are earthenware, crockery, enamel, or pyrex.

Unless the recipes state otherwise, hard substances, such as roots and barks, are prepared as decoctions (boiled continuously for a certain length of time), whereas soft substances, such as flowers, leaves, or blossoms, are prepared as ordinary teas (the herb or herb mixture placed in a cup or pan, boiling water poured on, and the tea allowed to steep). In each case, the container is covered with a lid until the boiling or steeping period is ended. If only one cup rather than a pint or more of the herb substance is steeped as tea, the cup is simply covered with a saucer.

2

CHINESE HERB REMEDIES FOR STOMACH DISORDERS

The word dyspepsia means to digest with some difficulty or pain. Indigestion may be a more old-fashioned term, but it means the same thing.

An estimated 30 million people in the United States suffer from chronic digestive disturbances. The usual causes of indigestion are wrong food combinations, eating too fast, drinking too much fluid with meals, not chewing the food properly, overeating, anxiety and nervousness, swallowing air while eating, and intolerance toward sugars, fats, and starches. The common symptoms are heartburn, sour belching, a heavy uneasy feeling in the stomach after a meal, headache, coated tongue, nausea, vomiting, flatulence, a bad taste in the mouth, foul breath, and sometimes difficult breathing and palpitation.

The Dangers of Non-Absorbable Antacids

Throughout the United States, sufferers from indigestion gobble up antacid tablets by the ton every day. An occasional antacid tablet to relieve stomach upset is harmless enough, but to take the tablets constantly, week in and week out, as some people do, is asking for trouble.

According to a medical report, a team of doctors found that phosphorus depletion results from the frequent use of antacids that are not of a dietary nature and cannot be absorbed. (Your bones are the "storehouse" for phosphorus, and when this mineral is inadequately supplied, your bones are in danger of becoming soft or brittle.) Many of the drug store patent antacid preparations available in tablet or liquid form contain either or both, magnesium hydroxide and aluminum hydroxide. Right here we'd like to point out that there is a great difference between magnesium hydroxide, which cannot be digested by human stomachs, and the fully absorbable magnesium mineral which occurs naturally in various foods and plants and is so valuable in human nutrition.

To quote the medical doctors who submitted the report: "It has long been known that non-absorbable antacids containing magnesium-aluminum hydroxides can bind gastrointestinal absorption of phosphorus." In their studies, phosphorus depletion was achieved in subjects by prolonged administration of antacids containing magnesium hydroxide and aluminum hydroxide. The doctors stated that in all subjects a number of striking events occurred, which included "a state of debility characterized by weakness, anorexia [loss of appetite], and malaise [a feeling of being ill]. In the patient A.S., severe bone pain and stiffness developed and persisted throughout the study. M.I., in addition, manifested an intention tremor of the hand . . ."

You Have a Choice

No doubt if you suffer from stomach distress you want to take something to relieve it. But why use indigestible forms of antacids that threaten to demineralize your bones and make you a very ill person indeed, when wholesome and digestible antacids are so easily available from natural herb remedies? Mother Nature is the true alchemist, and the precious treasures of her plant kingdom can neutralize the acidity gently, safely, and effectively.

A Word about Ulcers

It is estimated that one out of ten people will develop a duodenal ulcer at some time in their lives. This type of ulcer occurs in the short tube directly following the stomach. Some duodenal ulcers are very large—as much as four inches in diameter, while others are microscopically tiny.

Sufferers from duodenal ulcers may secrete as much as four times the amount of gastric juice in the empty stomach as normal persons. The pain of duodenal ulcer is often called "hunger pain" since it can be relieved by eating food.

The gastric type of ulcer occurs in the inside of the stomach area. Pain is felt in the stomach, and it also radiates upwards and to the back. It almost always starts shortly after a meal and produces a sort of burning sensation which is intensified by indigestible food, but relieved by a milk- diet.

A peptic ulcer simply means an ulcer occurring in the esophagus, stomach, or duodenum.

Many people carry an ulcer through life with nothing more serious than chronic annoyance, while some ulcers cause intense suffering and even death.

Chinese Herb Remedies for Stomach Disorders

Certainly medical doctors who employ surgery get good results in treating ulcers. Sometimes there is just no other way to save the patient's life. But when there is no real emergency, the ulcer victim may find relief through the use of natural Chinese herb remedies. The remedies are soothing and gentle, and many people have found them very effective. The same is true, of course, of specific Chinese remedies for coping with acid indigestion and other forms of stomach distress.

The natural ingredients called for in the recipes that follow are easy to use, easy to prepare, and easy on your pocketbook.

CHIEH-KENG

English Name: Chinese Bell Flower
Botanical Name: *Platycodon grandiflorum*

The decorative Chinese bell flower has a red stem, large dark-blue flowers, and smooth strong leaves. In China it is eaten as a pot-herb and considered very wholesome.

Medicinally, the plant is used for various ailments, but particularly for treating dyspeptic vomiting of mucus. It is also considered an excellent stomach tonic.

A decoction is made by slowly boiling two ounces of the cut roots in one quart of water for 15 minutes. The strained brew is taken in teacupful doses three to four times daily.

CHIANG

English Name: Ginger
Botanical Name: *Zingiber officinale*

Ginger is among the top-ranking botanicals in the Chinese materia medica. It is given for dyspepsia, loss of appetite, nausea, vomiting, and alcoholic gastritis. Chewing the root and swallowing the juice causes copious saliva to flow and stimulates the digestive juices. It is also chewed to relieve nausea and vomiting. Some professional Chinese cooks keep a small piece of ginger root in their mouth to prevent nausea from prolonged exposure to strong cooking odors.

The root prepared in the form of a tea improves sluggish digestion, relieves gas bloat, and stimulates the appetite. One-half ounce of the powdered root is stirred in one pint of boiling water, and two to three tablespoons of the tea are taken three times a day.

For upset stomach due to that morning-after "hangover," prompt relief may be obtained by sipping one or two cups of hot ginger tea for breakfast.

Chinese Ginger Remedy for Building a Healthy Digestion

The following remedy is reputed to be excellent for restoring strength and tone to the stomach and building a healthy digestion. The Chinese claim it is especially good during the cold weather as it has a warming and comforting effect on the stomach and is felt throughout the entire system.

Step 1. Put one-half cup of white rice in a flat bowl. Pour in enough water to barely cover the rice. Let stand overnight so that the rice can completely absorb the water. In the morning if there is any water still standing in the bowl drain it off. Put the rice in a dry frying pan, and gradually heat it until the pan is quite hot. Use a spatula, and keep turning the rice slowly so it doesn't burn. When the rice is parched dry and golden brown, put it in a glass jar and cap tightly against moisture.

Step 2. Bring one cup of water to a boil; add one teaspoon of the parched rice and a small piece of ginger root. Boil for one minute, and then turn off the burner and let stand for five minutes. Strain. Take one teacupful once or twice a day.

PO CHAI

Po Chai is a Chinese product made with several select herbs formed into tiny pills about the size of buckshot. The pills come in small phials, which are packed ten to a carton.

To thousands of Chinese-Americans, Po Chai is a well-known and proven remedy for the relief of acid indigestion, heartburn, and gas bloat.

Dosage: Adults—the contents of one phial. If necessary repeat in two hours. The pills may be swallowed with hot water or mild tea.

Woman Praises Po Chai

"I was raised near San Francisco's Chinatown," writes Mrs. T.L., "and had many wonderful Chinese-American friends. I learned to eat Chinese food with chopsticks, play the fascinating game of mah-jong, and even to speak a little of the language.

"One Thanksgiving Day, right after eating a sumptuous meal, mother and I dropped in for a visit with some of our Chinese friends. We hadn't been there 15 minutes before my mother began feeling ill. She complained of heartburn, a heavy feeling in her stomach, said that she was nauseated and couldn't seem to take a deep breath.

"I was alarmed, but one of our Chinese friends said, 'Too much turkey, pumpkin pie, and other rich Thanksgiving food,' while the others nodded in agreement. He took a small bottle of tiny herb pills out of the kitchen cabinet, gave the pills to my mother, and told her to take them with a glass of water. Ten minutes after she took the pills, she was feeling fit as a fiddle again.

"That evening before we left for home, mother wrote down the name of the herb pills. They were called Po Chai. From that time on we have followed the custom of our Chinese friends and have always kept a supply on hand as a stand-by home remedy for indigestion."

HUANG-LIEN

English Name: Gold Thread
Botanical Name: *Coptis teeta*

Among its many virtues, gold thread is considered an excellent bitter tonic for dyspepsia. It improves digestion, restores appetite, and relieves inflammation of the stomach lining. Gold thread is also employed to assist the treatment of alcoholism.

How to Use Gold Thread

The root may be used either in the form of a tincture or a decoction.

To prepare the decoction, place two ounces of the cut root in one quart of water, bring to a boil and simmer slowly for 20 minutes, and then strain. Dose: One tablespoonful four to six times a day.

To make the tincture, place one ounce of the cut root in a pint of good brandy. Cap tightly and allow to stand for one week, shaking the bottle once or twice a day. Strain. Dose: One teaspoonful in half a glassful of water three times a day.

HU-LU-PA

English Name: Fenugreek
Botanical Name: *Trigonella foenum-graecum*

The demulcent and carminative properties of fenugreek are considered valuable in relieving stomach gas and inflammation of the stomach and intestines. For any of these conditions, the powder is sprinkled over foods or a tea is prepared by adding one teaspoonful of the seeds to one cup of boiling water. The cup is covered with a saucer, and the tea is allowed to stand for 15 minutes, then strained. One cupful is taken three times daily.

Fenugreek is also employed for mild forms of peptic ulcers. The following account is but one of many examples of its effectiveness:

"I had a stomach ulcer for a great many years. It never bothered me so long as I stayed away from raw fruits, fruit juices, coffee, and meat. But I love these things, and every once in a while I couldn't resist the temptation to have some of them, and of course my ulcer let me know about it.

"Then I remembered that someone once told me of a Chinese herbalist who recommended fenugreek for stomach ulcers. I made a tea out of the powdered seeds, just like you make instant coffee, and drank one cup before each meal. Well, after three weeks of drinking the tea, I had a meal of my 'forbidden fruits' with absolutely no

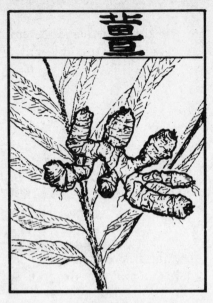

CHIANG
(Ginger)

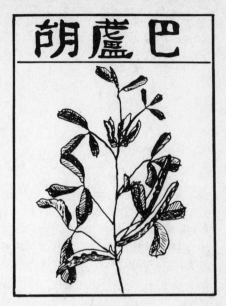

HU-LU-PA
(Fenugreek)

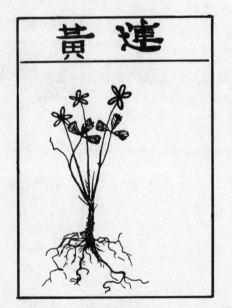

HUANG-LIEN
(Gold Thread)

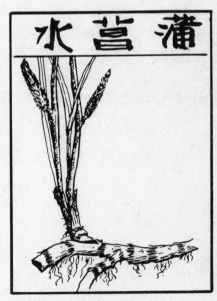

SHUI-CH'ANG-PU
(Sweet Flag)

stomach distress whatsoever. I continued to drink the tea for several weeks more. At the end, I found that I could eat anything I wanted."—Mr. T.P.

JENSHEN

English Name: Ginseng
Botanical Name: *Panax schinseng*

Ginseng tea is considered an excellent stomach tonic. One cup taken daily before meals stimulates the appetite, prevents sour eructions, and restores normal digestion.

Directions: Place the contents of one small envelope of powdered ginseng in a cup and add boiling water. These little envelopes are called "Instant Ginseng Tea" and are available from herb companies and health food stores.

HSUN-TS'AO

English Name: Melilot
Botanical Name: *Melilotus arvensis*

The name melilot is derived from the words *mel* (honey) and lotus, meaning honey lotus. The plant grows abundantly in the Yangtse region of China and contains aromatic and carminative properties.

A tea of melilot helps induce belching for the relief of gas bloat. The Chinese claim that it will also impart a lovely fragrance to the whole body.

Prepare as ordinary tea, and take one cupful three times a day.

SHUI-CH'ANG-P'U

English Name: Sweet Flag
Botanical Name: *Acorus calamus*

Sweet flag has long been credited with medicinal virtues both by ancient and modern Chinese herbalists. In olden times the herb was also regarded as a magical plant. On the Chinese New Year, Cantonese cleaned out their homes and posted the sword-shaped leaves of sweet flag near the door. Beneath them they placed a pair of red scrolls bearing an inscription such as "The sweet flag like a sword destroys a thousand evil influences."

Medicinal Use

Sweet flag is a specific for the type of heartburn that is accompanied by sour eructions. This is a distressing condition in which belching brings up from the stomach a hot, searing, watery fluid, sometimes in considerable amounts. For prompt relief a few small pieces of the cut root of sweet flag are chewed and the juice (not the roots) swallowed. This should be continued for five or ten minutes. In chronic conditions, the roots may be chewed several times a day until the stomach is back in good healthy working order.

If you prefer to drink the tea rather than chew the roots, mix one ounce of the powdered root in ten ounces of boiling water. The tea is taken warm, in doses of two ounces, twice or three times a day.

Case History

Mrs. J.G., a postal clerk, relates the following:

"For almost five years I suffered periodically from sour belchings, with all that terrible scalding water and sometimes even small pieces of food coming up in my mouth and throat. I tried all sorts of things that are supposed to help this particular condition, but they didn't help.

"One day a friend of mine told me that she was going to a Chinese herbalist for her rheumatism and about how much he was helping her. I made an appointment with him, and while there I began to have that miserable sour belching. I was frantic and asked the herbalist to please get me a glass of water.

"He left the room and quickly returned, but instead of bringing the water he handed me some small pieces of what he called sweet flag root and told me to chew them immediately and swallow the juice.

"I did as he asked. Almost at once, the terrible burning in my throat subsided, and in a matter of minutes my stomach quieted down.

"I took home a good supply of the roots and chewed the little darlings every day for a few weeks. That was over six months ago, and I have never had an attack of that horrible sour belching since. Isn't that remarkable?"

MI-TIEH-HSIANG

English Name: Rosemary
Botanical Name: *Rosmarinus officinalis*

According to tradition, rosemary was brought to China from the Roman Empire during the reign of Wenti of the Wei Dynasty.

Medicinally, the herb is used for nervous sick stomach, to clear the stomach of mucus, and to restore appetite and normal digestion.

Prepare as ordinary tea, add a pinch of ground ginger, and drink three or four cups daily.

CH'IAO-MAI

English Name: Buckwheat
Botanical Name: *Fagopyrum esculentum*

Buckwheat is very nourishing and digestible and has always been an important food crop in the central provinces of China.

Honey made from buckwheat has proven effective in some cases of peptic ulcers. Consider the following examples:

• Mr. R., a business executive, suffered from a duodenal ulcer for several years. Medical treatments helped for a while, but sooner or later the ulcer trouble always returned.

A Chinese herbalist told him to eat buckwheat honey and to use it in place of sugar as a sweetening agent. Mr. R. announced, "It's hard to believe that something so simple would prove so effective. Not only did it heal my ulcer, but taking the buckwheat honey daily, as I continue to do, has prevented any further recurrence of the trouble in over two years."

• Mrs. C.V., a housewife, writes: "With five children, an invalid father-in-law to care for, and a husband who is a chronic complainer, I wasn't too surprised when an X-ray showed that a small ulcer was forming in my stomach. I'm deathly afraid of any kind of surgery, and since food is one of the few pleasures in my life, I just couldn't face the thought of a milk diet.

"On the other hand, I knew that I had to do something or the ulcer might get progressively worse and I'd probably land in the hospital. So I got the idea to try a Chinese herbalist. He told me to take a teaspoon of buckwheat honey four or five times a day and to stay away from fried foods, bread, coffee, smoking, and alcohol.

"I don't know if this treatment would help everyone, but for me it was excellent. In less than a month the ulcer was healed. I still use the buckwheat honey daily as a preventative measure, and I can eat anything I want."

• A woman, age 30, took several spoonfuls of buckwheat honey every day during the hay fever season to prevent hay fever. When the season ended, she was astonished to find that a long-standing ulcer condition had cleared up.

• A salesman in his early forties suffered periodic bouts of ulcer pains. Buckwheat honey cleared up the ulcer, and he reports that he takes the honey daily as a preventative against any further trouble.

Buckwheat's Anti-Ulcer Power

Every effort is made by medical doctors to neutralize stomach acid, because the acid is highly irritating to ulcers. Honey is an alkaline food, and darker honeys such as buckwheat have a higher alkaline level than the lighter ones. Honey also provides many valuable minerals, and, interestingly enough, the mineral content is higher in those darker honeys.

Among its many constituents, honey contains magnesium, the spark plug which starts the chain reaction which metabolizes food. It is one of the richest sources of rutin, the nutrient so useful in strengthening the capillaries (tiny blood vessels). It also contains an anti-hemorrhage factor believed to be vitamin K.

Honey is assimilated rapidly and easily, and it is very soothing to the delicate membranes of the digestive tract.

WU-PA-HO

English Name: Peppermint
Botanical Name: *Mentha piperita*

Peppermint grows almost everywhere in China, but since the supply coming from Suchou is reputed to be of the best quality, the plant is called Wu-pa-ho, Wu being the former name for Suchou.

Peppermint tea has a delightful, comforting effect on the stomach and imparts a nice fragrance to the breath. Since it is carminative in action, one cup of the beverage after meals induces belching and therefore relieves the heavy distressed feeling of gas distention in the stomach.

For gas cramps, nervous upset stomach, nausea, or vomiting, one cup of the hot peppermint tea is sipped slowly every hour for three hours.

The tea is prepared by placing one teaspoonful of the leaves in a cup and adding boiling water. It is covered with a saucer to retain the aromatic properties, allowed to stand for five minutes, and then strained.

MU-SU

English Name: Alfalfa
Botanical Name: *Medicago sativa*

The reputation of alfalfa as an important healing agent for various ailments, including those of the stomach, can be traced back to the writings of the ancient Chinese. In an early Oriental herbarium, 896 plants are cited, and alfalfa tops the list. This herb originated in Persia and was allegedly brought to China by General Chang Chien of the Han dynasty.

Remarkable Plant

Alfalfa possesses deep feeder roots which burrow far into the earth, seeking out valuable minerals in the deep subsoil which are unavailable to other plants. Many instances are on record in which roots were found to have penetrated to depths of thirty-eight feet, while even greater depths of fifty to sixty-eight feet and over have been recorded.

This plant contains protein, calcium, phosphorus, iron, potassium, choline, sodium, silicon, magnesium, and eight essential enzymes. It also provides vitamins A, D, B_6, K, U, and P (rutin).

Alfalfa Used in Chinese Ulcer Treatment

Alfalfa tea is used to strengthen digestion and to stimulate a lagging appetite. It is prepared in the same manner as ordinary tea and taken freely as a daily beverage. Alfalfa also forms an important part of a Chinese remedy for stomach ulcers:
Directions:

- One tablespoonful of powdered alfalfa in a glass of water once a day.

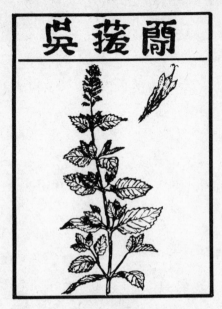

WU-PA-HO
(Peppermint)

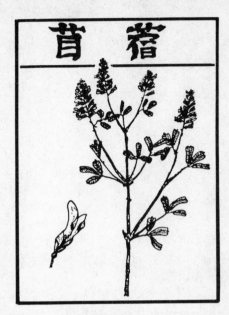

MU-SU
(Alfalfa)

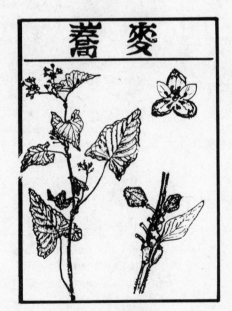

CH′IAO-MAI
(Buckwheat)

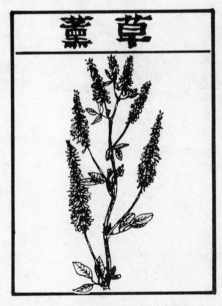

HSUN-TS′AO
(Melilot)

• One teaspoonful of olive oil before meals.

• Diet: No fried foods, no bread, no alcohol, and no smoking.

Interesting Case Histories

Here are some examples of sufferers who improved by using the Chinese ulcer treatment. These accounts were submitted by Mrs. V.C., who writes:

"I began having stomach pains, which proved to be caused by an ulcer. My doctor told me to start drinking milk, first half-and-half, and that later I would be drinking about three quarts of milk every day. I told him I was allergic to milk and cream, that they cause my asthma to flare up. He then suggested surgery, but the thought of an operation terrified me, so I politely left his office as quickly as I could.

"I decided to try a Chinese-American herbalist, but didn't realize how difficult it would be to find one. Finally I succeeded in doing so, but only by making a trip to one of the large cities in another state.

"The herbalist put me on alfalfa, one tablespoon of the ground powder dissolved in a glass of water once a day, and olive oil, one teaspoonful before meals. I was sure he would mention diet, and I was scared stiff it would be milk or cream and my whole trip would have been for nothing. So you cannot imagine how relieved I was to see that the diet did not stress dairy products. And it was such an easy diet, just no fried foods, no bread, and no smoking or drinking (I never drank or smoked anyway).

"The relief from the stomach pains was astonishingly prompt, and after I followed the treatment for a few weeks, my stomach ulcer had completely healed. This was not my imagination because I had my family physician check out the healing, and it was confirmed by X-rays.

"I have told many others who suffered from ulcers about this remarkable Chinese treatment, and they, too, have been helped. My brother was one. His doctor had him on a milk diet and bland foods, but the milk made him very constipated. He was terribly nervous and cross as a bear from the constipation, so after I told him about the wonderful results I got with the Chinese remedy, he stopped taking the milk and used my treatment. There was no more constipation or nervousness, and several weeks later his ulcer had disappeared.

"And then there was my neighbor. He tried the remedy, but

didn't like the taste of olive oil, so he dropped that part of the treatment and just followed the rest of it. And even though it took longer, his ulcer cleared up. Can you imagine that!

"I also told a lady friend about the Chinese ulcer treatment. The poor dear had been on a starvation diet for over a year and a half, and in all that time her ulcer had only partially healed. She told me that the thought of continuing the prescribed diet for much longer gave her a terrible feeling of despondency.

"She switched to the Chinese remedy and was delighted to find that she could eat more liberally with no distress. She told me, 'If the treatment did nothing more than allow me to eat better meals I would always be more than grateful.' So you can imagine how happy she was when, some weeks later, X-rays showed that her stomach ulcer was healed.

"I could go on and on about others who have also been very successful in using the Chinese treatment for their stomach ulcers."

Possible Clues to the Effectiveness of Alfalfa

Some of the elements contained in the Chinese ulcer treatment may offer important clues as to why many people have found the remedy effective. Let us examine these elements in the light of modern science.

Alfalfa. As we have seen, among its constituents alfalfa contains vitamins A, B, K, U, P (rutin), and eight important enzymes. Their therapeutic value is scientifically defined as follows:

- Vitamin A: Important for keeping the mucous linings of the stomach healthy.

- Vitamin K: Helps the blood clot properly and protects against hemorrhages.

- Vitamin U: This vitamin is known as the anti-peptic ulcer dietary factor. It is also present in cabbage juice and was discovered in 1949 by Dr. Garnett Cheney, a physician from Stanford Medical School. Dr. Cheney treated his ulcer patients with cabbage juice and found that 62 out of 65 of his patients responded in half the time necessary for the usual type ulcer therapy.

  Following Cheney, other reports on vitamin U studies began to appear. In 1954, George Kohler discovered that alfalfa was a good source of this important vitamin. In 1960, two German scientists studied the inhibitory effects of vitamin U on ulcer formation in dogs.

In 1971, after years of encouraging results from testing vitamin U on lab animals, Soviet scientists began clinical testing of vitamin U on human patients suffering from gastric and duodenal ulcers. To date, more than 1,000 patients have been treated. The therapy included five to six vitamin U pills daily for thirty to forty days. Results showed that whereas only 40% of ulcer patients are cured with the standard method of treatment, 80% were cured with vitamin U therapy and the remaining 20% were notably improved.

• Vitamin P (rutin): The appearance of an ulcer is generally preceded by inflammation of the stomach lining, and this in turn is the result of capillary weakness. Rutin is one of the bioflavinoids, and these natural substances reduce lining inflammation and build capillary strength.

Three medical doctors reported marked success with bioflavinoids in treating 36 cases of bleeding duodenal ulcers. In all 36 cases treated, the mucous membranes and duodenal contour returned to normal, usually in about three weeks.

• Enzymes: According to Dr. Jacobson, food scientist of Reno, Nevada, there is a sufficient quantity of enzymes in alfalfa to be of considerable aid in the digestion of all four classes of food—starches, proteins, fats, and sugars.

Olive Oil. It is well known that olive oil has a soothing effect on the lining of the stomach. Devett Fox, M.D., treats his ulcer patients with olive oil and reports that it does the same or an even better job than the cream given in traditional ulcer diets. Some medical doctors have speculated that olive oil contains vitamin U, the ulcer healing substance.

The Chinese Ulcer Diet

You will notice that the Chinese diet is not the traditional ulcer diet prescribed by orthodox medics. This is very impressive, since a number of modern medical experts conceded years ago that there is very little advantage in the standard milk-heavy, bland ulcer diet, and recently the editors of *Drug and Therapeutics Bulletin* have reaffirmed these opinions.

The *Bulletin* says that a diet of steamed fish, milk, and purees over a long period of time is apt to cause a patient to suffer from iron and vitamin C deficiency, plus complications of diarrhea, gas, and constipation. If the patient has surgery, he is especially cautioned to avoid the traditional ulcer diet afterwards.

The *Bulletin* adds that the patient who eliminates fried foods, stops smoking, and stops heavy drinking is taking sensible anti-ulcer action.

SUMMARY

1. Symptoms of indigestion may appear as heartburn, sour belching, gas bloat, foul breath, flatulence, nausea, vomiting, headache, coated tongue, bad taste in the mouth, and sometimes palpitation and difficult breathing.
2. There is a distinct possibility that frequent use of antacid preparations containing magnesium or aluminum hydroxides can render the bones more fragile than they ought to be.
3. Natural Chinese herb remedies can do the job of neutralizing stomach acids safely and effectively.
4. Many other forms of stomach distress can also be relieved by wholesome, select Oriental plant remedies.
5. Specific Chinese herb formulas have coped effectively with some cases of peptic ulcers.

3

CHINESE HERB REMEDIES
FOR RESPIRATORY AILMENTS

According to Chinese herbalists, there are a large number of specific plant remedies that can deal effectively with various ailments of the respiratory tract. These natural healing agents help fight infection, reduce fever, loosen stubborn phlegm, soothe inflamed air passages and linings, make breathing easier, and bring an end to dragged out respiratory miseries that cause considerable suffering.

If you are badgered by colds, sore throats, or other infections or ailments of the respiratory tract, you may find Chinese herb remedies of great benefit. However, please remember that nature demands cooperation, which means proper diet, rest, and clean living habits.

YIN-HSING

English Name: Ginko Tree
Botanical Name: *Ginko biloba*

The name "Ginko" comes from the Chinese and means "silver fruit" or "white nuts." This tree grows abundantly south of the Yangtse and in other regions of the Far East, but has also been cultivated in Europe and the United States. The fruits are highly prized in the Orient, and the roasted pits are considered a delicacy.

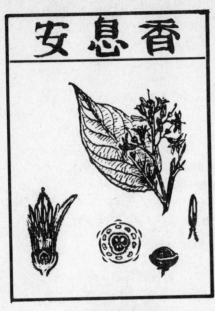

AN-HSI-HSIANG
(Gum Benzoin)

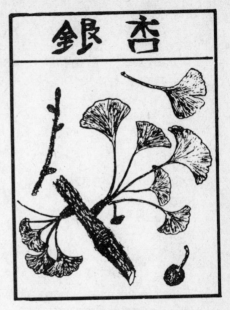

YIN-HSING
(Ginko)

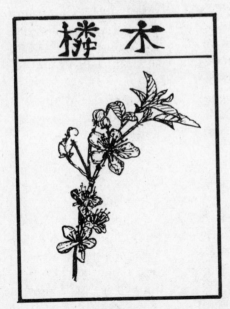

LIN-MU
(Wild Plum)

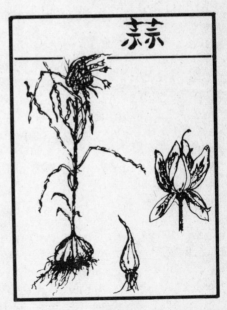

SUAN
(Garlic)

In our own country, however, the fruits are rarely seen on the Ginko because the staminate and pistillate flowers occur on different trees and usually only the staminate types are planted.

Centuries ago, the Ginko was found growing in a courtyard of a Chinese temple, and it has since been classified as one of the oldest living species of trees. Today the Ginko is familiar to tree lovers everywhere, not only because of its great beauty, but also because it has a peculiar and mystifying immunity to insects and diseases which attack other trees. Even though its remarkable resistance to such pests has made the Ginko a horticultural curiosity, scientists have yet to discover what substance in the tree imparts the immunity. The Ginko is also very tolerant of dust and city smoke and is not usually damaged by storms.

A Specific for the Common Cold

The Chinese have long claimed that the leaves of the Ginko contain medicinal properties that can cure the common cold very quickly and that these properties are also effective in relieving sinus congestion, stubborn coughs, and asthma. For any of these purposes, the leaves are infused in boiling water and the vapors from the steam inhaled.

Those who may be skeptical of the Chinese claim for the Ginko as a curative remedy for the common cold may want to hesitate in their criticism and ponder the following report.

According to a German newspaper, Dr. Joachim H. Volkner, a nose, ear, and throat specialist in Berlin, announced the discovery of a "lightning" cure for the common cold. Dr. Volkner found that if a person inhales an essence prepared from the leaves of the Ginko tree, his cold will get better. Two hundred and twenty-four people tried the Ginko treatment, and the results were "staggering." The German report stated that, "The inflamed areas healed immediately."

Dr. Volkner confesses that he hasn't as yet identified the exact substance in the Ginko leaves that produces the therapeutic effects, but he does explain how the treatment works. When a person catches a cold, the cells of the mucous membranes are damaged and are unable to store moisture. The efficiency of the cell walls becomes impaired because substances in the cell press against these walls. Apparently, the Ginko essence forces these components of the cell back into its interior. Dr. Volkner explains that "The microbes which have collected inside die off, and very shortly after inhalation [of the Ginko essence] they completely disappear."[1]

PIEN-HSU

English Name: Knotgrass
Botanical Name: *Polygonum aviculare*

Pien-hsu (knotgrass) is a low-growing herb which has been used in China as a remedy for lung ailments since the second millenium B.C. The Chinese often call the plant Fen-chieh-ts'ao because of the white powder that covers the stem.

Along with tannin, mucilage, and small amounts of volatile oils, knotgrass contains salicylic acid, a powerful pharmaceutical agent which no doubt accounts for the herb's long-standing reputation as a remedy for lung diseases. In modern Chinese medicine the plant is employed for treating bronchitis and whooping cough. It is prepared as a tea, one teaspoonful of the cut herb to one cup of boiling water. Three to four cups of the strained infusion are taken daily.

K'UAN-TUNG

English Name: Coltsfoot
Botanical Name: *Tussilago farfara*

K'uan-tung is commonly known in Western countries as colts-foot or coughwort. The botanical name, *tussilago,* signifies "cough dispeller." Some of the Chinese names refer to the herb's early flowering and its resistance to cold and frost.

Nature's Cough Remedy

Coughing helps you to eject excessive mucus or food particles and other foreign material that interferes with your breathing. However, when the mucus deposits are stubborn and very deep-seated the cough persists. And it may also persist when the lungs are irritated due to smoke, dust, or infection, even though there is no material to eject. This is the type of cough that gives you that aggravating "tickle."

---

[1]*Hamburger Abendblatt,* October 8, 1966.

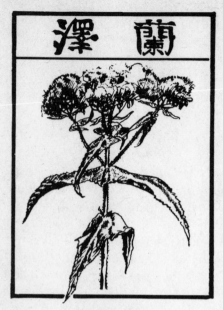

TSE-LAN
(Boneset)

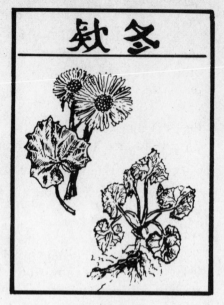

K'UAN-TUNG
(Coltsfoot)

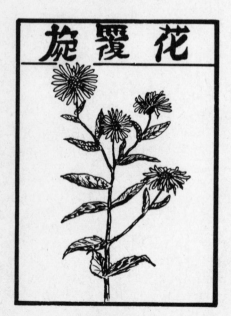

HSUAN-FU-HUA
(Elecampane)

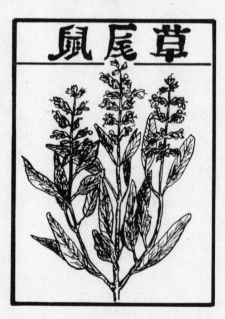

SHU-WEI-TS'AO
(Sage)

It is important to take every possible step to reduce the severity and persistence of coughing so that you can get your sleep and proper rest. The experience of Chinese herbalists has shown that a tea made of coltsfoot leaves and other select herbs is very helpful for relieving stubborn coughs and irritations of the lungs and air passages. The formula consists of the following:

K'uan-tung (coltsfoot leaves) . . . . 1 oz.

Hu-lu-pa (fenugreek seeds) . . . . 1 oz.

Chiang (crushed fresh ginger root) . . . . ¼ oz.

Put the fenugreek seeds and ginger root in one quart of cold water and bring to a boil. Simmer for 10 minutes. Strain. Pour the boiling decoction into a container in which one ounce of coltsfoot leaves has been placed. Mix well, cover, and allow to stand until cold. Strain, reheat, and add one tablespoonful of honey and a small amount of powdered Kan-ts'ao (Chinese licorice root). Three to four cups of the tea are taken daily for irritable cough, wheezing, or throat irritation.

PEI PA KOA

English Name: Loquat Syrup

Loquat syrup, a translation of the Chinese language pronunciation of the name Pei Pa Koa, was originated by Kingto Nin Jiom in the Ching dynasty. This herb formula has a fascinating history. According to the story, which is reportedly true, Governor Yeung of Peiping (the city where the King lived) was extremely filial to his mother and terribly grieved because she suffered frequent attacks of painful sore throat and severe coughing spells. Many famous doctors were consulted, but none were able to help.

Then one day Governor Yeung heard of a learned Chinese physician named Yip Tin Sie and immediately engaged him to cure his mother's illnesses. This wise doctor bethought himself of the formula originated by Kingto Nin Jiom and decided to treat her with the herb syrup. After Governor Yeung's mother fully recovered, the doctor gave Governor Yeung the secret formula for the syrup and told him how to prepare it. The Governor was further instructed to give his mother some of the syrup twice a day, once in the morning and once in the evening, to maintain her health and to prevent any further recurrence of her ailment.

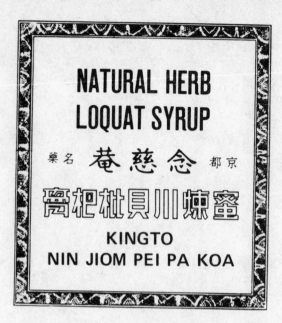

Front Label of Loquat Syrup

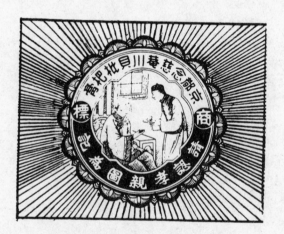

Section of the Loquat Syrup label
showing Governor Yeung giving the
herb remedy to his beloved mother.
Note the yin-yang motif of the
circle—half white and half black.

48

Governor Yeung was so grateful for his mother's recovery that he prepared bottles of the syrup and gave them away free to anyone who suffered from the same illness.

After the Governor's death, the demand for bottles of the syrup became so great that his descendants were forced to charge a little money for them, but to every bottle they attached the complete formula and the mark and words "Filial To Mother Device" in honor of their ancestors.

The gesture of revealing the exact contents of the precious formula is quite amazing since the Chinese, especially long ago, went to great lengths to keep the ingredients of their remedies a carefully guarded secret. For example, they would hire blind people to roll the herb ingredients into pill form or other forms, so that no one aside from the herbalist himself could possibly know what the formula contained. Thus, by revealing the ingredients of the Loquat Syrup, Governor Yeung's descendants certainly performed a humanitarian act.

Pei Pa Koa Comes to the United States

Pei Pa Koa (Loquat Syrup) contains absolutely no chemicals of any kind. It is a purely natural formula containing eleven herbal ingredients, and it is still prepared in the traditional method.

This syrup, which has been used for centuries in China, is now imported into the United States, and many people are claiming excellent results with its use. One young man who suffered from weak lungs and coughing spells for over a year reported that the syrup worked for him where orthodox medicine had not. He said, "I really didn't think the Chinese herb syrup would do much more than bring me a little relief, but after taking it every day for several weeks I was entirely free of my chronic lung trouble." An elderly woman reported that the use of the syrup cleared up a stubborn condition of nasal congestion. In another case, a man wrote: "Constant tickle of 'smoker's cough' yielded entirely with the use of Loquat syrup, and I found the same to be true of an aggravating cough due to a bad cold."

HSUAN-FU-HUA

English Name: Elecampane
Botanical Name: *Inula chinensis*

This plant is native to North China, Manchuria, Mongolia, and Korea and appears to be the same as *Inula britanica,* the English elecampane. Other Chinese names for the plant are Chin-ch'ien-hua and Chin-ch'ien-chu, applied generally to the cultivated variety which resembles the herb *calendula.*

Sometimes the whole dried plant—including the leaves, roots, flowers, and stalks—is found on sale in Chinese herb shops. However, the root is the part chiefly used in Chinese medicine.

The medicinal action of elecampane is cited as diaphoretic. It is used in combination with other specific herbs for the relief of bronchitis, hay fever, and asthma.

For example:

Hsuan-fu-hua (elecampane) . . . . ½ oz.

Han-t'ao (cherry bark) . . . . ½ oz.

Sung (white pine) . . . . ½ oz.

Ch'ien-hu (angelica root) . . . . ½ oz.

Kan-ts'ao (Chinese licorice root) . . . . ¼ oz.

Place the herbs in one quart of boiling water; boil slowly down to one pint, strain, and add honey to make a syrup. One table-spoonful is taken four times a day or more often if the cough is very troublesome.

The Chinese claim for elecampane as an important remedial ingredient for various respiratory ailments has received some scientific support. It was established that inulin, the chief constituent in the plant, is a powerful antiseptic and bactericide especially destructive to the tubercule bacillus.

LIN-MU

English Name: Wild Plum
Botanical Name: *Prunus spinulosa*

The flowers of the wild plum are single or in pairs and are very small compared to those of the domestic or garden plum. The wild species grows in Central China and Europe and appears in our own country in the double flowered variety.

The antispasmodic action attributed to wild plum bark is said to be of considerable value for treating asthma. Place one teaspoon of the cut, dried bark in one cup of boiling water, cover, and allow the tea to stand until cold. Strain, reheat, and add a little honey. Dose: One cupful one hour before meals three times a day.

Following are some interesting reports on the use of wild plum bark tea:

• "I am using wild plum bark tea before bedtime and upon arising for asthma and bronchitis. It certainly has been helping me. I have given this a long trial and can testify to the wonderful help received. Of course, right living and eating has also aided materially."—Mrs. S.B.

• "I have spent a small fortune on medicine for asthma in the last three years, and with no results. I heard about wild plum bark and purchased a supply, and I have been able to sleep from the first night on."—Mr. B.Y.

• "I want to tell you what the good wild plum bark has done for me. I have suffered for fifteen years with asthma, and this spring I was down for 12 weeks. Three doctors could not help. One of my neighbors, a Mrs. J.G., ordered some wild plum bark, and it put me on my feet in a week. I certainly can never say enough for it."—Mrs. R.V.

TIGER BALM

Tiger Balm is a popular Oriental herb ointment developed more than a half a century ago by two Chinese brothers, Aw Boon Par and Aw Boon Haw. Aw is the surname, Boon means "gentle," and Haw means "tiger," so the brothers decided to call their formula Tiger Balm.

This Chinese herb product comes packed in three sizes—large jars, medium jars, and small tins. It also comes in two colors, red and white, and in two strengths, mild and strong. The jars and tins containing the stronger formula, called Red Tiger Balm, are wrapped in a reddish-pink paper, whereas those of the milder product, White Tiger Balm, are wrapped in white paper.

Remedial Benefits of Tiger Balm

Tiger Balm relieves tightness of the chest and produces a soothing effect on the pains due to colds, fatigue, exposure, strain, or rheumatism. For such conditions the parts are well rubbed with the Chinese ointment two or three times a day and covered with a warm flannel.

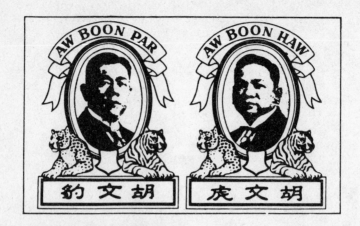

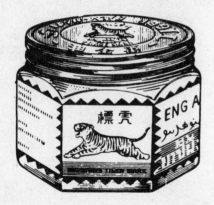

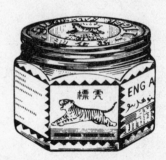

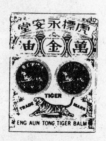

TIGER BALM
Medical Ointment

Tiger Balm is also used as an inhalant for stuffed up noses, nasal drip, and head colds. A few whiffs of the vapor soothes the upper air passages and gives your head a clear feeling.

Some Interesting Reports on the Use of Tiger Balm

• "For years I have suffered from sinus congestion with very little relief. Then I heard about Chinese Tiger Balm. Dabbing a little of the ointment under each nostril and inhaling the vapors brought such relief that I will never be without it."—Mrs. R.B.

• "Inhaling the fumes from the open jar of Tiger Balm is the only thing that has given me relief from the discomfort of hay fever."—Miss P.M.

• "Whenever I get neuralgia pains I use Tiger Balm. It relieves the pain considerably." —Mrs. V.S.

• "I had the flu, and my muscles and bones ached so badly I couldn't sleep. My wife bought a jar of Chinese Tiger Balm, which worked like magic. And we found that Tiger Balm is good for other things too. My sister was troubled with nasal drip and had to carry a packet of Kleenex in her purse at all times. At our suggestion, she agreed to try Tiger Balm. Two days later we got a phone call from her. 'I could kiss you both,' she said. 'That Chinese product is absolutely marvelous.' "—Mr. T.P.

BALASHIN SAI
(Pat Kwa Tan)

Balashin Sai is another famous herb formula developed by the two Aw brothers. The active ingredients of this Oriental product are Gambier, peppermint oil, and Chinese licorice powder. These ingredients are compressed into tiny square lozenges which are used for the relief of coughs, colds, catarrh, sore throat, and nausea. Balashin Sai also sweetens the breath, counteracts perspiration odor, and serves as a refreshing stimulant for exhaustion.

• Mrs. J.R., a department store clerk, writes: "All my life I have suffered miserable spells of catarrh. Sometimes the aftermath of a cold or poor diet is the triggering cause. Other times I can not detect the cause. Getting to sleep at night was a dreadful chore because I'd be constantly trying to clear my throat to keep from choking on the phlegm. During the day, frequent clearing of my throat while serving store customers was terribly embarrassing.

Sai. They
are so effective and so easy to use. I simply put a few of the tiny
pellets on my tongue and let them dissolve slowly. The catarrh soon
clears up."

• The following comes from Jim R., a hard-working auto
mechanic: "At least once or twice a year I catch a cold that isn't
serious enough to keep me home in bed, but the scratchy sore throat
and dragged out feeling really get me down. These bouts have never
been any picnic for my wife and kids either because my disposition
goes sour.

"One of our neighbors told my wife about a Chinese herb
product called Balashin Sai and explained what the lozenges were. At
my wife's insistence, I used them. The soothing effect on my throat
was out-of-this-world, and I also experienced quite a refreshing
pickup, no longer had that lousy dragged out feeling. Hope you'll
pass the news of this Chinese remedy along to others."

HSIEH-TZU-TS'AO

English Name: Chinese Nettle
Botanical Name: *Urtica dioica*

Following is one of the specific remedies used by Chinese
healers for treating the condition of pleurisy.

Boil two ounces of dried Chinese nettles (or the seeds) slowly in
one quart of water for 20 minutes. Strain when cool, reheat, and
take one teacupful every two hours. In addition, apply hot fomentations to the painful side. For this purpose prepare a second quart of
the nettle decoction. Dip a flannel in the hot tea, wring out and place
on the affected part, cover with a dry towel, and retain until cool.
Then renew the flannel, and continue the hot fomentations until
relief is obtained. Chinese herbalists have reportedly cured many a
severe case of pleurisy with the above treatment.

CHANG

English Name: Camphor
Botanical Name: *Cinnamomum camphora*

This is an evergreen tree of great size, which produces red
berries much like cinnamon. The Chinese name, Chang, is said to be

derived either from Yu-chang, an ancient name for Kiangsi, where the tree grows abundantly, or from Chang-chou-fu in Fukien, where large quantities of camphor are produced.

Camphor has been made in China since the earliest periods and was already well known to Chinese writers in the sixth century. Marco Polo saw many camphor trees when he visited that country, and Camoens in 1571 called the tree "the balsam of disease." During the process of extracting camphor an oil exudes which is highly prized by Chinese herbalists, who credit it with many medicinal virtues.

A Favorite Stand-By Remedy

Among the Chinese, camphor and camphorated oil are used externally as anodynes (pain relievers) and counter-irritants for muscular aches and pains, chest congestion due to colds, and other inflammatory conditions. The soothing vapors from a solution prepared by placing small pieces of gum camphor in boiling water are inhaled to clear nasal stuffiness caused by head colds. For fever sores a little camphor is applied directly and frequently to the sore. For the relief of simple colds warm camphorated oil is rubbed on the chest, back, and over the bridge of the nose.

Bottled camphorated oil can be purchased from drug stores, or the oil can be prepared in your own home by dissolving one ounce of finely powdered camphor in four ounces of warm bland oil such as soybean oil or olive oil.

Camphor Remedy for Bronchitis

Chronic bronchitis is a long-standing disease of the bronchial tubes. Coughing and shortness of breath often accompany this debilitating ailment, and when the condition persists, emphysema may result.

For two years, a junior high school boy suffered from chronic bronchitis, and the usual agents prescribed by orthodox medics for this condition did not help. The desperate parents finally took the boy to a modern Chinese-American herbalist. They were told to purchase a heat lamp and a good supply of camphorated oil. Each night at bedtime the oil was to be rubbed gently, slowly, and continuously over the boy's chest for 20 minutes, while at the same time shining the heat lamp on the chest area close enough to throw a good heat, but not so close as to cause a burn. When the 20 minutes were up, the same treatment was to be used on the lad's back.

The parents applied the treatment faithfully for several weeks, after which time their son was entirely free from any symptoms of bronchitis. Today he is a grown man with children of his own and has never had a recurrence of the debilitating ailment.

TSE-LAN

English Name: Boneset
Botanical Name: *Eupatorium perfoliatum*

Tse-lan (boneset) is an important ingredient of a Chinese formula for colds, catarrh, and especially for influenza symptomized by fever, headache, aching muscles, and pains in the bones and joints. Generally after four or five doses have been taken profuse sweating occurs and relief is obtained:

Tse-lan (boneset) . . . . ½ oz.

Wu-pa-ho (peppermint leaves) . . . . ½ oz.

Chieh-ku-mu (dried elder blossoms) . . . . 1 oz.

Simmer the elder blossoms in one pint of water for 20 minutes, then strain. Place the boneset and peppermint leaves in a separate container and add one pint of boiling water (do not allow the infusion to continue boiling). Cover, allow to stand for one-half hour, and then strain. Add this brew to the elder tea, and then reheat the mixture and drink one-half pint hot every 15 minutes until relief is obtained.

Note: There are different species of elder. The one cited in this formula is known botanically as *Sambucus canadensis.*

AN-HSI-HSIANG

English Name: Gum Benzoin
Botanical Name: *Styrax benzoin*

A medicinal aromatic gum resin is obtained from an Asiatic tree called *Styrax benzoin* and is imported into Southern China from Sumatra and Borneo. The "An-hsi" in the Chinese name, An-hsi-hsiang, probably refers to the Persians, whose country, along with Sumatra and Central Asia, is a source of supply for this foreign balsamic resin. The aromatic resin is obtained by making triangular cuts in the bark of the tree. From these incisions exudes the sap which coagulates, and after it has sufficiently hardened it is collected and packed for export.

At one time in China, the fumes resulting from burning this lovely smelling substance were believed to drive away devils and attract good spirits.

Benzoin for Croup

The active ingredient of the gum resin is extracted and made into a tincture called "benzoin." This valuable tincture is universally used, both in Chinese and orthodox medicine, as an inhalant for dry, hacking coughs, those which doctors call "unproductive." This is a condition in which it is extremely difficult to cough up apparently immovable sputum from the bronchial tubes. It is commonly known as "croup."

Any mother whose infant has had the miserable ailment of croup knows how terrifying it is to watch the feverish child desperately trying to cough up the obstructive phlegm. For such emergencies, benzoin tincture is reputed to be of great value. One teaspoonful of the tincture is added to one pint of boiling water. Under a sheet arranged like a tent, the vapors from the mixture can be inhaled by the youngster. This loosens up the unproductive sputum, much to the great relief of the croupy child and the alarmed mother.

Laryngitis

Laryngitis is an inflammation of the larynx (voice box). Symptoms include hoarseness, irritation, difficulty in breathing (you wheeze), and frequently a dry, rasping cough. Your voice may be reduced to a mere whisper, break into a high falsetto pitch, or descend to a deep bass. Talking is very uncomfortable, and if you overuse your voice the laryngitis condition may become serious.

The benzoin inhalation method outlined for treating croup may also be used by adults suffering from laryngitis. Steam from one-half hour to one hour four times a day.

Along with recommending the steam inhalation, Chinese herbalists suggest that you take it easy, drink plenty of liquids, and spare your voice as much as possible. They also point out that laryngitis is aggravated by temperature changes, so you will recover more quickly if you stay at home when you have this ailment.

KAN-TS'AO

English Name: Chinese Licorice
Botanical Name: *Glycyrrhiza glabra*

Kan-ts'ao (Chinese licorice) grows abundantly in Northern China, and quantities are also brought from Mongolia, especially from the region of Kokonor. Other names for the plant are Mi-kan, Mi-ts'ao, Mei-ts'ao, Lu-ts'ao, Ling-t'ung, and Kuo-lao. The last name cited is applied because of the herb's great virtues as a remedy.

Licorice root is considered to be of great importance in Chinese pharmacy, being the corrective and harmonizing ingredient in a large number of prescriptions. In Chinese herb shops the root is commonly sold in long, dry, wrinkled pieces.

Demulcent, pectoral, alterative, emollient, expectorant, and slightly laxative properties are attributed to Chinese licorice root. It is used to relieve thirst, feverishness, coughs, hoarseness, sore throat, and distress in breathing. The extract enters into the composition of cough lozenges, syrups, and pastilles.

- For irritable cough, scratchy sore throat, or laryngitis, boil two ounces of licorice root in one quart of water until reduced to one and a half pints. Add one ounce of K'uan-tung (colts-foot leaves) and two tablespoons of lemon juice to the simmering decoction, and immediately remove the container from the burner. Keep the brew covered and allow to stand until cold. Strain, reheat, and drink one cup of the hot tea three or four times a day.

- The following formula lubricates the throat, loosens stubborn phlegm, and affords relief in hoarseness, coughs, and bronchial irritations:
    Kan-ts'ao (licorice root) . . . . ½ oz.
    Chih-ma (flaxseed) . . . . 1 oz.
    Boil in 1½ pints of water for 10 minutes, then strain. Dose: One cup of the hot tea, three or four times a day. Sip the tea slowly.

SUAN

English Name: Garlic
Botanical Name: *Allium sativum*

Suan (garlic) has been known to the Chinese from earliest times and was mentioned in the Calendar of the Hsia, a book written two thousand years before Christ. According to Chinese tradition, when the Emperor Huang-ti was climbing a mountain some of his followers ate the leaves of a poisonous plant and became deathly ill. By eating wild garlic which was also found growing in the area, their lives were saved. From that time, the bulb was introduced into cultivation.

Garlic—a Valuable Remedy

No doubt you are quite familiar with the little garlic bulb as something which you use to flavor your steaks, stews, roasts, and salad dressings. But according to Chinese herbalists, if you have garlic in your kitchen, you have what comes close to an all purpose healing agent. They claim that the common little bulb acts as a wide spectrum antibiotic without side effects, and that it also possesses many other medicinal virtues. For example, it is used in conditions of asthma, bronchitis, colds, diarrhea, autointoxication, pin worms, abscesses, nervous indigestion, and much more. However, we shall limit our attention here to the Chinese usage of garlic in treating respiratory ailments.

Colds—Coughs—Asthma—Bronchitis

1. For the treatment of colds, coughs, sore throat, hoarseness, asthma, and bronchitis, the freshly expressed juice of garlic is well mixed with honey, and a teaspoonful of the mixture is taken at repeated intervals. (In conditions of bronchitis, bread is eliminated from the diet.)

2. A stronger garlic syrup may be prepared by pouring a pint of boiling water over two ounces of finely chopped garlic. This is kept in a closed container and allowed to stand for 10 hours. It is then strained, a tablespoon of Ts'u (vinegar) is added, and the preparation is mixed with enough honey to form the consistency of a syrup. This mixture is a strong expectorant for conditions of deep-seated coughs, dry hacking coughs, and chronic bronchitis.

3. Garlic tea is another preparation used for treating stubborn coughs and colds and is also said to relieve sinus trouble. Either the fresh garlic cloves or garlic in powder form may be employed for making the tea. Add one-quarter teaspoon of

the powder to one small teacup of hot water. Sip one teacupful slowly, three or four times a day.

If preparing the tea from fresh garlic, place two to four freshly chopped garlic cloves in a saucepan and add one quart of boiling water. Steep as ordinary tea, strain, and sip one hot cupful three or four times a day. If the cough or cold is very severe, the tea may be used every hour until relief is obtained.

Many people have reported excellent results from using garlic tea. For example, Mr. C.W. relates the following experience.

• "I caught a very bad cold which settled in the bronchial tubes, and I coughed constantly day and night. Neither drug store cough syrups or patent medicines did any good. Doctor's prescriptions didn't help either. Luckily, I spotted a small paragraph in a newspaper which said that Chinese herbalists often advise garlic for respiratory ailments.

"I stirred a little garlic powder in a small glass of hot water and drank it down slowly. My cough lessened almost immediately. For one week I continued taking the garlic tea about three or four times a day, sometimes more often, after which time all my cold symptoms were gone."

• Another interesting report comes from Mrs. J.W., who prepares her garlic tea from the fresh cloves.

"When our children get runny noses, coughs, nose bleeds, or just colds in general, I make garlic tea and give it to them quite hot. Next day they have no stopped up heads. This is also good for sinus headaches. I repeat this every hour for sinus trouble and pneumonia."

4. For whooping cough or colds that affect the chest, one part freshly expressed garlic juice is mixed with two parts soybean oil, and the mixture is rubbed on the chest and back every night before you retire. This external application is generally used in conjunction with any appropriate internal garlic remedy cited in this chapter.

5. Daily doses of garlic taken in any suitable way is another method credited with fighting diseases of the nose, throat, and lungs. Asthma, bronchitis, whooping cough, colds, catarrh, nasal congestion, pleurisy, and seizures of prolonged sneezing are examples.

• One woman suffered an attack of almost continuous sneezing, as rapid as 15 per minute, for six days. She was given a diet of fresh garlic (plenty of chopped garlic in soups, salads, and so on), which halted the seizures for several hours, but the attacks resumed again in moderate form the next day. The garlic diet was continued, and the seizures subsided and finally ceased.

Tonsillitis

Two ounces of Shu-wei-ts'ao (sage) and one tablespoon of fresh garlic juice are added to one quart of boiling water. The preparation is covered, removed from the burner, and allowed to stand until luke warm. It is then strained, and one small teacupful is taken four or five times a day. The complete treatment consists of preparing another quart (or more) of the sage-garlic tea for use as a hot gargle, one cupful every half hour.

Nasal Congestion

Place a little chopped garlic and one teaspoon of T'su (vinegar) in one pint of boiling water and inhale the fumes. Repeat as often as necessary.

Protective Power of Garlic

Chinese healers believe strongly in preventative medicine and rate garlic as one of the best protectives against various respiratory ailments. Many years ago in Manchuria, during pulmonary plagues, the Chinese people ate large quantities of garlic to help guard themselves against infection.

As a protective agent, garlic may be taken daily in tablet or capsule form, or a fresh clove or two can be eaten, a few small pieces at a time, throughout the day.

Two Classic Examples of Garlic's Protective Power

1. Every day Mrs. Y.W. gave her four-year-old daughter a garlic tablet to nibble on. Two months later, Mrs. Y.W. decided to spend a week's vacation with her sister who lived in another state. Upon her arrival, she was alarmed to find that all three of her sister's children had whooping cough, even though they had been innoculated against the disease. For one week Mrs. Y.W.'s own little four-year-old

daughter was exposed to a constant barrage of whoops, yet the child did not catch the disease.

2. "We have just completed another mind-expanding sojourn to three Latin American countries—Colombia, Ecuador, and Panama. Once again we took our garlic capsules each day (5 grain extract of garlic in vegetable oil sealed in gelatin capsules) and had no sickness. We did not stay at the usual tourist haunts, but traveled into the most primitive sections of these countries. We ate everything put before us and drank their water. We literally followed the philosophy of 'when in Rome, do as the Romans do.' We visited the villages of Indians who, just a matter of a few years ago, were killing Christian missionaries, and who are now baptizing their children and following the way of the Lord, primarily as the result of the work of Wycliffe Bible Translators in these countries. We were exposed to all the diseases common to them, but our garlic held forth . . .

"We heartily recommend garlic capsules for those Americans who plan on traveling to different countries, particularly when the water and food are often contaminated."—Prof. H.L.M., Jr.

Tuberculosis

Many Chinese healers credit the following treatment with being effective in conditions of tuberculosis.

In order to purge the body of poisons, the patient is instructed to keep the bowels open and to eat fresh garlic in any suitable way, starting with one ounce the first day and gradually increasing the amount each day until by the end of the week three or four ounces can be taken daily. This amount is continued each day until the purgation period is over, and then it is gradually reduced to one ounce daily for three months.

The patient is also instructed to place finely chopped fresh garlic in boiling water and to inhale the fumes for two or three minutes several times a day. A bottle of garlic extract may be used by simply removing the cap and inhaling the fumes periodically. In addition, the chest and back are rubbed with a mixture of garlic juice and soybean oil every night just before the patient goes to sleep.

Westerners Agree with Chinese Claims for Garlic

Some people of other lands have found that this garlic treatment can be applied with some slight variations and still be equally effective. For example, here is one woman's remarkable account of what garlic did for her:

"I had been confined in a Western hospital for about seven years with tuberculosis . . . a new nurse appeared . . . After the nurse heard my problem, she said, 'Many people have been cured in my home town.' She said reassuringly, 'When you arrive home get about two pounds of garlic into the house and keep plenty of it on hand. Take one ounce of peeled garlic daily, preferably between meals, chop it finely, crush it, and eat it in a cupful of soup, in carrot juice, or in some other vegetable juices. Whichever way you take it, do so gradually until at the end of the week you will be getting three to four ounces daily. By then the poisons will start eliminating from the body so that you will think you will die—but you won't. In advanced cases it may take about three to four weeks before the purgation is complete, then one tapers off until only one ounce daily for three months is consumed. During the purgation period it is well to assist the cleansing process by drinking all the liquids possible between meals (no coffee or tea at any time). Vegetable and fruit juices are recommended. Avoid mixing because some fruits and vegetables do not harmonize and can create gases in the intestinal tract. In the morning and before retiring at night, take enemas after each bowel movement. This will aid in elimination and help in building new villi and capillaries. Also, you can put finely chopped garlic on a piece of paper and, while resting, inhale its odor for minutes at a time. No matter how people may ostracize you, just continue using it until your whole bloodstream changes and throws off the poisons the disease has manufactured inside you. In about three months time you will be able to do chores around the house, and you will grow strong enough in a short time to lead a normal life.'

"I followed the nurse's instructions to the letter, and as my husband did not object, I ate garlic in every way I could think of—with green string beans, diced carrots, and so on. I would cut up a clove of garlic, add it to the boiling liquid two or three minutes before turning off the fire, and then add two teaspoonfuls of soy or olive oil, and eat it with the liquid. I prepared cream cheese with chopped celery or parsley leaves and then mixed garlic with some. I crushed it and mixed it with French dressing and used it over all vegetable salads. Anyone may prepare other kinds of soup.

"During the purgative period my body eliminated such black mucus and 'sick' liquid, I could hardly believe it was inside me. With the aid of fruit and vegetable juices and daily enemas, after about four weeks time my bowel excrement became normal and life seemed worth living again.

"When I went to the hospital for a check up, the orthodox doctors did not recognize me. Neither would they believe me when I told them about the 'cure.' One remarked, 'Nothing like that has ever been used.' X-rays, however, gave me a clean bill of health despite their belief."

Supportive Evidence of Chinese Claims for Garlic

Modern medical evidence supporting the claims by Chinese herbalists that garlic is an effective remedy for tuberculosis and other respiratory ailments can be seen from the following reports.

• Christine Nolfi, M.D. states that garlic can successfully handle many diseases of the respiratory tract. She says this applies to colds and also "to chronic inflammation of the tonsils, salivary glands and neighboring lymph glands, empyema of the maxillary sinus, severe pharyngitis and laryngitis, bronchitis, and tuberculosis of the lungs." Dr. Nolfi also informs us that, "At Humlegaarden (a health sanatorium) epidemic colds are unknown. Everyone knows that he must use garlic when a cold begins. Since a cold may develop into pneumonia in the case of weak patients, it is better avoided."

• In an article written in the *New York Physician,* H.E. Kotin, M.D. and David Stein, M.D. tell of their experiences in treating their patients with garlic. Twelve case histories are cited, and these cases ranged from tuberculosis to asthma, bronchitis, shortness of breath, chills and fever, pharyngitis, and so on. Every single case obtained relief in one month, some in one week.

• Dr. Minchin, an English physician in charge of a large TB ward at Kells Hospital, Dublin, published reports on the successful treatment of tubercular consumption by the administration of garlic as an inhalant, an internal medicine, and as compresses and ointments. He found that garlic has a specific destructive action on the bacillus of tubercle in human patients. Many doctors in all parts of the world were keenly interested in Dr. Minchin's reports.

• In an article entitled "Tuberculosis Treatments," Dr. M.W. McDuffie tells of 56 different treatments that were used on 1,062 tubercular patients. Of the 56 treatments employed, Dr. McDuffie says: "Garlic is the best individual treatment found to get rid of germs, and we believe the same to be a specific for tubercule bacillus and for tubercular processes no matter what part of the body is affected. Thus nature, by diet, rest and exercise, baths, climate, and garlic, furnishes sufficient and specific treatment for medical aspects of this disease."

CHINESE HERB GARGLES AND MOUTH WASHES

Germs that trigger colds, tonsillitis, influenza, and similar ailments generally gain access by the mucous membranes of the mouth and throat. As an accessory treatment to the various plant remedies previously covered, Chinese herb gargles and mouth washes are of great value since they remove germs from your mouth and throat, and help speed your recovery.

These natural herb solutions are also helpful for treating canker sores, mouth ulcers, ulcerated gums, bleeding gums, and similar conditions.

Beneficial for Oral Hygiene

When you are exposed to chilly winter months or a barrage of sneezing and coughing, infection may hover all around you, but the full force of the attack may be repelled if you indulge in a melodious herbal gargle or mouth wash every morning before going to work and before going to bed at night. Along with their protective powers, these herbal preparations build mouth and gum health and also modify unpleasant odors that linger in the mouth after certain meals or beverages.

Directions for Use

Some of the Chinese recipes cited in the following list are used solely for treating a specific condition of the mouth and throat, while others may be used either as a treatment or for daily oral hygiene.

For treatment purposes, an herb gargle or mouth wash is used four times a day, or more often if necessary. In conditions of sore throat, tonsillitis, and similar ailments, herb gargles are more effective if used as hot as possible, but not so hot that they burn. Mouth washes are used warm or cool. For bleeding gums, the herb preparations are used cold.

For daily oral hygiene, a mouth wash or gargle may be employed once in the morning and once again at night, or you may clean and rinse your mouth with the herbal solution whenever possible after eating. When you use an herb gargle for daily oral health, it should be used warm, not hot.

MU-YAO

English Name: Myrrh
Botanical Name: *Balsamodendron myrrh*

From remote antiquity, the fragrant gum-resin of the myrrh tree has been a constituent of Oriental medicines, perfumes, incense, precious ointments, and sacred oils. Originally imported from Persia, the gum-resin of myrrh is now produced to some extent in the southern regions of China.

As a mouth wash, one-half teaspoon of myrrh tincture in a glass of warm water soothes delicate mucous membranes of the mouth and throat. It is also very soothing and healing for troublesome canker sores, denture irritated gums, or when gums are sore from rough brushing or sensitive from dental work. The lovely aroma and flavor of myrrh tincture imparts a lasting, refreshing taste and fragrance to your mouth and breath after strong flavored foods. Try it also every morning to refresh your mouth after that stale overnight taste and mouth odor.

Tincture of myrrh may be applied full strength to cold sores.

HUANG-LIEN

English Name: Gold Thread
Botanical Name: *Coptis teeta*

Huang-lien (gold thread) is used as a gargle or mouth wash for minor sore throat, canker sores, and irritation of the mouth due to smoking. It is also used warm for aphthous sore mouth in children (a condition symptomized by many small white blisters in the area of the mouth and throat).

Boil two ounces of the cut roots of gold thread in one quart of water for one-half hour. Strain, and add one teaspoon of honey.

SHU-WEI-TS'AO

English Name: Sage
Botanical Name: *Salvia officinalis*

Sage was so highly regarded by the Chinese that they gave the early Dutch traders twice the amount of their choicest Oriental teas in exchange for it.

This herb is an aromatic astringent and an antiseptic of subtle and penetrating power. It is used alone or in combination with other herbs.

- Place two ounces of sage in a container and pour one quart of boiling water over them. Cover with a lid, remove from the heat, and allow the tea to stand for two hours. Strain, and add one tablespoon of honey and a tablespoon of Ts'u (vinegar). Use as a hot gargle for stubborn sore throat or inflammation of the tonsils.

- Simmer one ounce of sage in one pint of water for ten minutes, then allow it to stand until cold. Strain, add a teaspoon of honey, and use as a hot gargle for throat irritation or cool as a mouth wash for ulcerated mouth and ulcers or bleeding of the gums. Excellent for use in daily oral hygiene as it increases the resistance of the mucous membranes to infection. As an added bonus, this sage tea is reputed to be of great help to public speakers because it strengthens and sustains the voice. One tablespoon of the tea is swallowed just before you go to the meeting.

- For the condition of tonsillitis, prepare a strong sage tea, two ounces to one quart of boiling water. Remove immediately from the heat, cover, and allow to stand for two hours. Strain, and add a small bit of pulverized alum.

  One woman who tried this sage-alum gargle wrote: "My oldest boy got up with tonsillitis one morning, so I prepared a tea of sage and alum and had him gargle with it several times a day. The next day he was rid of the tonsillitis, where other times he would suffer for weeks and could not eat or sleep."

- Here is another formula Chinese herbalists often prescribe for tonsillitis: Place one ounce of sage and one ounce of Chin-ssu-ts'ao *(Hypericum chinensis*—a species of St. John's Wort) in a container and add one quart of boiling water. Cover, and allow the tea to stand for one-half hour. Strain, and add one teaspoon La-chiao (ground capsicum). Reheat, and gargle with it frequently.

- For the throat ailment of quinsy, prepare a quart of strong sage tea. When it is strained, add one teaspoon of ground La-chiao (capsicum) and gargle frequently.

Fomentations are also used in conjunction with the gargle. To one quart of strong sage tea, add one tablespoon of Ts'u (vinegar). Dip a cloth in the hot tea, wring out, and bind around the throat, using a dry towel over it to retain the heat. As soon as the cloth begins to cool, replace it with a fresh one and repeat the hot fomentations several times. Repeat throughout the day as often as necessary.

Chinese herbalists also advise that soups heavily seasoned with La-chiao (capsicum) should be a part of the diet to help put a more speedy end to quinsy.

HSIA-KU-TS'AO

English Name: Self-Heal
Botanical Name: *Prunella vulgaris*

This plant contains astringent and styptic properties and is used as a cold mouth wash for bleeding gums or as a gargle or mouth wash for ulceration or inflammation of the mouth and throat. Prepare a tea by adding one ounce of the leaves to one pint of boiling water. Remove from the heat, cover, and allow to stand for ten minutes. Strain.

PIEN-HSU

English Name: Knotgrass
Botanical Name: *Polygonum aviculare*

A strong tea prepared from Pien-hsu held in the mouth for five minutes relieves toothache and arrests bleeding gums. Prolonged use is said to harden loose, spongy gums, make the teeth less sensitive, and help prevent tooth decay.

Place one ounce of the herb in a saucepan and add one pint of boiling water. Cover and allow to stand until cold. Strain.

FAN-PAI-TS'AO

English Names: Cinquefoil
Botanical Name: *Potentilla reptans*

In ancient China, cinquefoil was used in magic for casting spells and as a love-divining herb.

Cinquefoil makes a fine gargle or mouth wash. Chinese herbalists employ it for its astringent properties to arrest bleeding gums and to fasten loose teeth. Used as a daily mouth wash, it builds strong healthy gums.

Place one teaspoonful of the herb in a cup and add boiling water. Cover with a saucer and allow the tea to stand for 30 minutes. Strain.

HU-CHIN-TS'AO

English Name: Violet
Botanical Name: *Viola odorata*

The violet plant contains salicylic acid, mucilage, resin, sugar, an aromatic principle, a glucoside, and an alkaloid. It is also a rich source of vitamins A and C.

A gargle or mouth wash prepared from violet leaves is used for inflammation, swelling, and ulceration of the mouth and throat and is also reputed to relieve the pain of cancerous growths, especially in these areas.

Fresh violet leaves are more potent; however if they are not easily obtainable, the dried may be used. Prepare as a strong tea, six ounces of the leaves to three pints of boiling water. Cover tightly, remove immediately from the heat, and allow the infusion to stand for twelve hours. Strain. Use as a gargle or mouth wash and, in addition, drink one small teacupful of the brew every two or three hours.

The reputation of the violet plant as a means for relieving the pains of cancer is fairly widespread. For example, when Catherine Booth, wife of the founder of the Salvation Army, was dying from cancer, an appeal was made for violet leaves since they alone could ease the agonizing pain. And of special interest are the studies of Dr. Jonathan Hartwell of the Cancer Institute of the National Institutes of Health. In citing the violet, Dr. Hartwell says: "The violet plant, as far back as 500 B.C., was used in poultice form as a cure for surface cancer. It was used in the 18th century in England for the same purpose. And now only months ago, a letter from a farmer in Michigan tells us how he used the violet plant as a skin cancer remedy. When the remedy was tried on a cancerous mouse here at the Institute, we found that it did damage the cancer . . ."

SUMMARY

1. Select Chinese herb remedies loosen stubborn phlegm, reduce fever, fight infection, soothe irritated air passages and lungs, make breathing easier, and help bring an end to dragged out respiratory miseries.
2. Garlic is a powerhouse of disease-fighting agents that make it an effective healer and preventative of various respiratory ailments.
3. Persistent coughing is very debilitating since it causes sleepless nights and distressing days. The remarkable properties of specific Chinese herb formulas can relieve your coughing miseries and enable you to get your proper sleep and rest.
4. External herbal applications relieve chest tightness and muscular aches and pains due to colds.
5. Select herbal inhalants are soothing and healing to the air passages. They are very helpful for coping with nasal congestion, head colds, croup, nasal drip, and similar conditions.
6. Chinese herb gargles and mouth washes are important accessory treatments because they remove germs from your mouth and throat and help speed your recovery. They are ideal for oral hygiene since they build mouth and gum health and increase resistance of the mucous membranes to infection.

4

GINSENG—CHINESE HEALTH HERB

Plaudits for Ginseng

For thousands of years the oldest civilization on earth has insisted that the root of a plant known in the Far East as Jenshen (ginseng) is the remedy *par excellence* for preventing or treating an incredible variety of ailments—and further, that it contains near miraculous powers which build energy and zest, sharpen the vision, improve hearing, increase the efficiency of the brain, restore virility, and prolong life. Other Oriental peoples have always fully agreed with the Chinese claims for ginseng, but it took an extraordinarily long period of time before the people of Western lands bothered to give these claims a second thought. Over the years missionaries in China, old-time family physicians, writers, and others tried to stimulate an interest in the Oriental usage of ginseng, and these attempts continued to grow.

• The late Sir Edwin Arnold, famed student of Oriental philosophy and author of *The Light of Asia,* wrote: "According to the Chinese, Asiatic ginseng is the best and most potent of all cordials, stimulant tonics, stomachics, cardiacs, febrifuges, and above all, will best renovate and reinvigorate failing forces. It fills the heart with hilarity, while its occasional use will, it is said, add a decade to human life. Have all these millions of Orientals, all these many generations of men who boiled ginseng in silver kettles and praised heaven for its many benefits been totally deceived?"

71

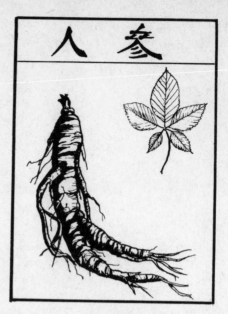

JENSHEN
(Ginseng)

• Some decades ago, a United States Consul of Korea submitted an official report stating: "From personal experience and observation I am assured that Korean ginseng is an active and strongly healing medicine. Western people appear to regard the virtues of ginseng claimed by Orientals rather contemptuously—as imagination or based on superstition. The evidence is that the mystical value attached itself to ginseng after its virtues had been practically ascertained."

• In his field notes, Father Jartoux, a missionary in China, described ginseng as an invigorator, rejuvenator, and longevity plant.

• S.E. Zemlinsky, author of a book on the medical botany of Russia, wrote: "Ginseng is not only a very popular Chinese medicine for longevity but is used in all parts of Asia. Its use is to prolong life, youth, virility, and health."

• A former Vice-Consul in Korea stated: "As to the merits of Korean ginseng, the Chinese at any rate had no doubts. Where vitality was becoming extinct from age or strength had been reduced by long illness, ginseng was employed with equal faith and success."

• Early in the century, Dr. A.R. Harding tested the Chinese claims for ginseng and reported that, much to his astonishment, he found that no matter what ailments his patients suffered from, they recovered more quickly when taking ginseng than when any other medication was given.

• The late Dr. H.S. McMaster wrote: "Ginseng is a mild nonpoisonous plant, well adapted to domestic as well as professional uses. The medicinal qualities are known to be a mild tonic, stimulant, nervine, and stomachic. It is especially a remedy incident to old age."

Growing Habits

Asiatic ginseng grows wild in deep shaded mountain forests of the Far East. It shuns direct and heavy sunlight, and its leaves are uniquely arranged to receive only a weak amount of light evenly. While other plants gather their nutrients in the root, leaves, flowers, and buds, the nutrients of ginseng are concentrated mainly in the root. At one time it was believed that ginseng could not be cultivated, but today we find that it is successfully grown in many lands.

More Precious Than Gold

During various periods of Chinese history, ginseng was worth many times its weight in gold. Sometimes an emperor would send an ounce or more of the root to a distinguished friend who was suffering from a serious ailment that had not yielded to other medications.

Usually the gift included a small double kettle for preparing the precious ginseng. The inner kettle was made of silver, and the outer kettle was made of copper. Between the two there was a space for holding water. Cut ginseng root and water were placed inside the silver kettle, and a small amount of rice and water was placed in the cup-like cover of the silver vessel. The kettle was then set on a ring which circled the top of the outer copper vessel, and the space between the two kettles was filled with water. The apparatus was then placed on the fire.

When the preparation was ready, the patient ate the rice and drank the ginseng tea at the same time. Usually the patient took the formula every morning before breakfast and sometimes in the evening for about eight days. Ordinary tea was forbidden for one month.

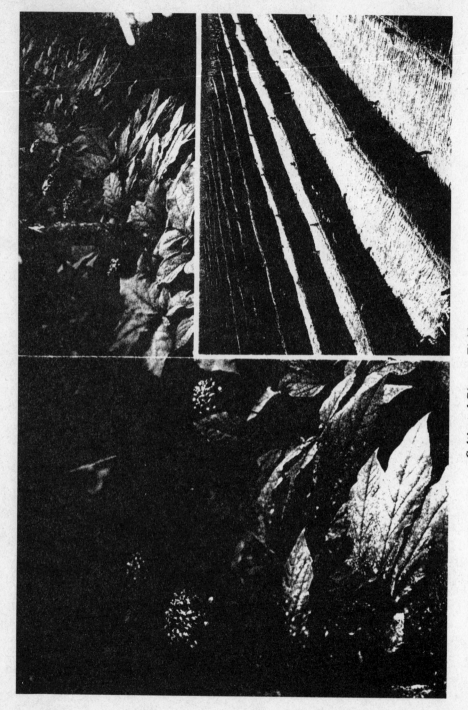

Cultivated Ginseng Field.
Inset shows slats which provide shade.

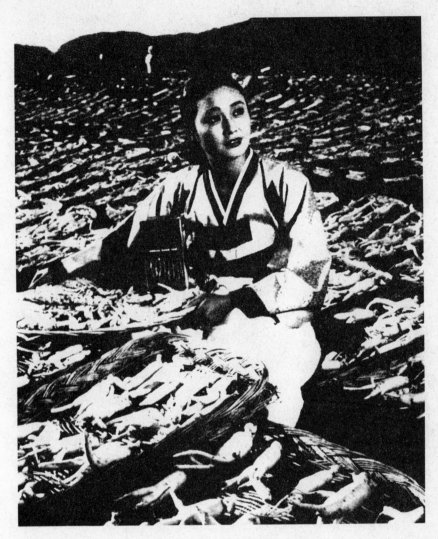

Raw Ginseng Roots Drying in the Sun.

Ginseng Synonyms

It is interesting to note that the many synonyms which the Orientals have attached to ginseng indicate the herb's traditional use or the high esteem in which it is held—Long Life Root, Man's Health, Queen of the Orient, Root of Life, Promise of Immortality, Divine Herb, Wonder Root, Flower of Life, Wonder of the World, and Man-Plant. The latter synonym actually refers to the shape of the root, which sometimes resembles the form of the human figure. Because of this resemblance, the Chinese composed the name ginseng from two words meaning "man-plant," and many Oriental legends refer to this human-like form of the root.

Ginseng in Modern Times

Today, in the space age, ginseng root is still widely used among Oriental peoples, and now, at long last, the popularity of the plant is rapidly spreading to other lands. In the publication *New Scientific Discoveries in Regeneration,* we read:

> The latest discovery from China is ginseng, the rejuvenation herb, considered by the Chinese as a panacea of all diseases. It is believed by its enthusiasts that ginseng overcomes disease by building up general vitality and resistance, and especially by strengthening the endocrine glands, which control all basic physiological processes, including the metabolism of minerals and vitamins.

The life span of former Korean President Syngman Rhee, who died at the age of 90, was attributed by Koreans to his long use of ginseng. Generalissimo Chiang Kai-Shek, the former leader of Nationalist China, was said to be a regular user of the long-life root. Madame Nhu reportedly took along a supply of ginseng on her trip to New York back in 1963.

In Australia ginseng is used to remedy a number of different ailments and to help perpetuate youthfulness and prolong life. The Russians use it to build mental strength, general vitality, and resistance and to treat various disorders. Some years ago, Dr. Finn Sandburg of Switzerland said, "Whenever I am in Singapore I have lunch with Han Suyin, author of *A Many Splendored Thing* and other best selling novels. As Elizabeth Comber, M.D., she practices medicine in Johore Bahru, near Singapore, prescribing mostly European and American drugs for her patients, but when she is sick herself, the only remedy she uses is ginseng root."

Ginseng in the United States

In the United States, a 23-year-old student, working hard on his thesis for a degree, told his friends, "I took ginseng last May and I never felt any fatigue this summer."

Another student found that smoking marijuana caused his memory to become sluggish. He quit smoking pot, but three months later when his memory still hadn't shaped up he consulted a Chinese herbalist. The herb doctor put him on ginseng, stating that it is an effective brain tonic and that it also acts as an antidote to certain types of toxic drugs. After taking ginseng extract for six weeks, the young student happily reported that his memory was better than ever.

In another case, a man 73 years of age was troubled with nervousness, indigestion, and brain fag. After a two months course of ginseng, he became calm, more mentally alert, and was no longer bothered by stomach distress. He says he continues to take the ginseng tonic to retain the benefits.

A 75-year-old woman complained of cold hands and feet, general debility, pains in the bones, depression, and memory lapses. She took ginseng for one month and noted some improvement. Encouraged, she continued taking the herb preparation and after four months her symptoms completely disappeared.

Celebrities Laud Ginseng

Even many of the movie and TV stars are reportedly using ginseng. In an article, "How the Stars Stay Forever Young and Beautiful," Peter Lupus, handsome, swashbuckling TV hero, is quoted as saying: "I brew it [ginseng] into an acceptable tea. I consider it a rejuvenator, an invigorator, a reactivator, and it's also supposed to be a good aphrodisiac. But one thing you must remember, you can't just brew one cup and swallow a capsule and say, 'Man, now I feel great!' A studio pal tried it for two days, reported he didn't see any difference in how he felt. You have to keep on taking it. You can't expect to use it for a week and see a miracle."

The article also quotes a movie actress in her early fifties: "I've been using it [ginseng] for months, since I was in Paris where I bought a face cream at $25.00 a jar and found it contained ginseng. When I asked about it, I was told that wealthy Oriental women drink ginseng tonics and tea, and they have gorgeous wrinkle-free skins. I decided to try ginseng as a tea, and I'm delighted with its effect on my skin. It stimulates me, removes the effects of fatigue, and seems to be helping me keep from catching colds."

Another movie star who was interviewed on the use of ginseng said, "I'm adding a teaspoon of ginseng tonic to my pre-dinner cocktail in place of bitters. I figure this should about average out—the ginseng will prolong my life about as much as the alcohol in the cocktail will shorten it. Yesterday my agent phoned me with some wonderful news about a lead in a film that will net me a pile of dough. I told him to hold the phone while I ran to get my ginseng tonic. The agent thought I was out of my mind! I told him I had to have a swig of my life-prolonging tonic. If I'm going to have that kind of money I want to be around to enjoy it as long as I can."[1]

Scientific Evaluation of Ginseng

Although ginseng is still largely ignored by most Western scientists, intensive pharmacological and clinical investigations of the Oriental root have been carried out by Soviet scientists. Many ginseng studies have also been undertaken by other qualified researchers covering such countries as China, Korea, Japan, and Germany. A special Ginseng Committee combining the efforts of all Russian scientists and practical workers engaged in this field has been in operation since 1949 and is subordinate to the Far Eastern Center of the Siberian Division of the USSR Academy of Sciences. During these past many years, the Committee held 23 sessions in which Soviet and foreign scientists participated. The Committee published seven volumes of works and a two volume collection of the minutes of the Committee sessions.

To briefly summarize, the results of these intensive studies have established that ginseng relieves atherosclerosis, acts as an antidote to various types of drugs and toxic chemicals, produces a good effect in a number of disorders of the central nervous system, helps to normalize the blood pressure and various other bodily functions, favorably affects the activity of the sex glands, protects the body against radiation, stimulates and improves the work of the brain cells, increases physical stamina and endurance, has an anti-rheumatic effect, improves vision and hearing acuity, and is a good adjuvant in diabetes mellitus, diseases of the liver, impotence, and several other diseases.

Dr. I.I. Brekhman, one of the leading scientists of the Soviet team, says that although the list of diseases in which ginseng is effective may be a long one, the root is not a panacea, a "cure-all." He explains that, "Ginseng, being a good tonic, a roborant, increases the resistance of the organism and helps it to overcome many

---

[1]Block, Maxine, "How the Stars Stay Forever Young and Beautiful," *Rona Barrett's Hollywood,* May, 1970, p. 23.

diseases of various origins." He adds that ginseng strengthens almost the entire bodily defense mechanism and refers to this fortifying power of ginseng as a "universal defense action."[2]

Research by Soviet and other foreign scientists has established that ginseng is harmless and acts only by improving physiological processes. "No bad effects are observed after taking it," the report states.

Ginseng and Longevity

The "universal defense action" of ginseng in preventing or treating a wide variety of ailments may be one of the reasons for the herb's traditional reputation as a longevity plant. Scientists tell us that disease is one of the principal causes of premature aging and a short life span. A list of some 90 diseases was submitted to a number of prominent physicians, along with a request to indicate the percentage of deaths from those illnesses which could have been prevented. Calculations based on returns showed that through a possible timely prevention, more than a dozen years could have been added to life.

Another factor believed by scientists to be partly responsible for the symptoms of aging is the gradual decline in the output of sex hormones that usually begins in the middle years of life. In youth these glands are healthy and active and are directly related to the general health and to the prolonged appearance of youth. If the sex glands are nourished, the precious hormones would once again be produced at higher levels similar to those produced by younger people. In short, the new supply of hormones would help delay the symptoms of old age. Soviet researchers have reported that, "Ginseng favorably influences the functions of the endocrine glands, in particular the hypophysis cerebri, the adrenal cortex, and the genital [sex] glands."

Several Varieties of Ginseng

There are several varieties of ginseng. To mention a few, the Chinese and Korean ginseng is known botanically as *Panax schinseng,* the North American variety as *Panax quinquefolium,* and the Japanese variety as *Panax japonica.* The generic name *Panax* is taken from the word for panacea, meaning "cure-all."

---

[2]Lucas, R., *Ginseng The Chinese 'Wonder-Root'* (Spokane, Washington: R & M Books, 1972), p. 40.

Koreans describe the various grades of their ginseng in poetic terms. For example, the Red Korean Ginseng roots are graded as follows:

Whole Roots
Heaven Grade (1st class)
Earth Grade (2nd class)
Good Grade (3rd grade, called Man-Grade)
Tails
Big Tail
Middle Tail
Scrap Tail
Slender Tail

The term "tails" refers to the smaller root divisions that grow out from the main body.

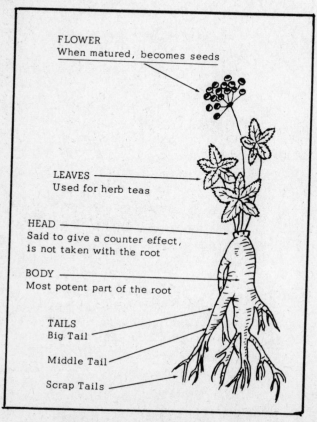

FLOWER
When matured, becomes seeds

LEAVES
Used for herb teas

HEAD
Said to give a counter effect,
is not taken with the root

BODY
Most potent part of the root

TAILS
Big Tail

Middle Tail

Scrap Tails

Different Parts of the Ginseng Plant

Available in Many Forms

Korean ginseng root is available on the market in many forms—whole, cut, bulk powder, powder in capsules, fluid extracts, tea bags, concentrated fluid extracts, and tiny envelopes of powdered instant ginseng. (There are also ginseng compounds and blends, but these are included in the following chapter.)

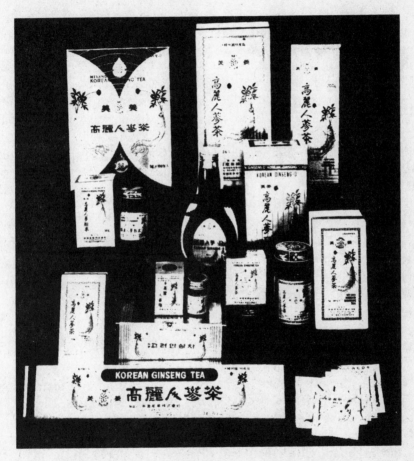

An Assortment of Various Ginseng Teas and Products

The only way to find out which particular form of ginseng root is best for you is to give it a fair trial. Ginseng is not a synthetic drug, it is a harmless yet potent natural herb. Directions for using the various ginseng products are listed on the labels. However, individual differences of each person should be considered. For example, some people may find they need greater amounts in order to obtain the benefits, while others find that smaller amounts are sufficient. And a few people may find that if they take ginseng just before going to bed, its stimulating properties tend to keep them awake. This is remedied by taking the preparation earlier in the day.

Further Tips on Ginseng

For best results, acid fruits, acid fruit juices such as orange, grapefruit, and so on, and vitamin C should be avoided for three hours after taking ginseng since they neutralize the beneficial effects of the herb.

If you decide to try ginseng, be sure to purchase your supply from a reliable firm. There have been instances where partially developed roots, stringy fibres, or "culls" of ginseng were shipped into this country. Linda Clark, nutritionalist, reported one such case where the owner of a store and his assistant used ginseng faithfully every day, but saw no benefits. The product they were using turned out to be a "cull" of some ginseng from which most of the strength had been removed before it was shipped to the U.S.

SUMMARY

1. Ginseng has a long history of usage among Oriental peoples for treating disease, preventing illness, and prolonging life.
2. Extensive research on ginseng by modern scientists, covering such countries as Russia, Korea, Japan, and others, has established that many of the Chinese claims for the therapeutic power of ginseng root are true.
3. Whereas the nutrients of many other plants are distributed throughout the leaves, roots, stems, flowers, and buds, the nutrients of ginseng are mainly concentrated in the root.
4. Ginseng is not a synthetic drug, it is a natural herb.
5. There are many different forms of ginseng available on the market. The only way to find out which form is best for you is to give it a fair trial.
6. For best results, acid fruits, acid fruit juices, and vitamin C should be avoided for three hours after you take ginseng.
7. If you decide to use ginseng, deal only with a reputable firm.

5

ORIENTAL HERB TONICS AND BLENDS

There are a number of Oriental herb blends and compounds available on the market which bring good results as healing agents or health tonics according to many people who have used them. These specially processed formulas generally consist of the main principal herb or root and several assistant and related herbs or roots or other natural substances. In addition, there are also a number of herb tonics which can be prepared right in the home.

As space does not permit a comprehensive listing of all the various compounds, tonics, and blends, only a few examples will be cited.

JIN SAM JUNG

This is a bottled extract containing a Korean ginseng root, ginseng extractive, honey, and royal jelly. The merits of ginseng have already been discussed, so let us briefly consider the nutritional value of honey and royal jelly.

Honey

It is well known that honey is a quick source of energy. Edward Bach, M.D. always advised his patients to eat honey to relieve tiredness and exhaustion.

In ancient times, many people believed that the regular use of this natural substance insured health and longevity. Modern studies

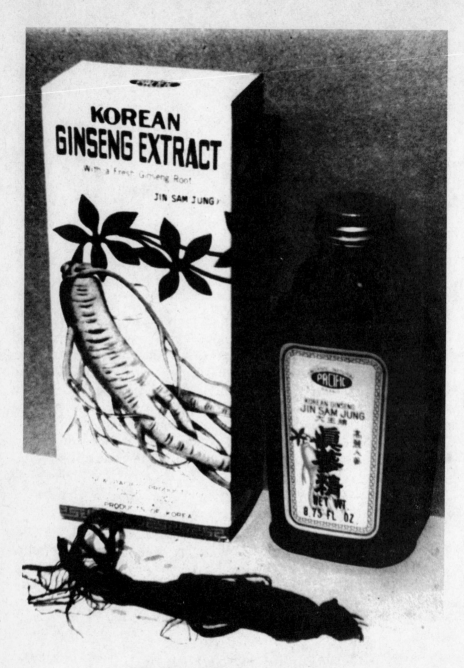

JIN SAM JUNG
Each bottle contains a fresh whole
ginseng root immersed in the extract

have shown that honey is an excellent tonic and reconstructive for convalescents, dyspeptics, and the aged. Because of its lubricating action, honey has a gentle and slightly laxative effect. Some medics have reported it to be a good heart tonic and also to be helpful for relieving nervous insomnia.

Royal Jelly

Royal jelly is a substance produced by young worker bees which is fed to the larva from which the queen bee develops. The queen rules the hive and receives royal jelly throughout her life. She performs an incredible amount of work and may lay as many as one-quarter of a million eggs in one season. Worker bees (no royal jelly for them) perform industriously for two to six months then die, but the queen bee lives as long as eight years. Experiments with royal jelly on animals have resulted in greater resistance to infection. The egg-laying capacity of hens fed royal jelly increased from 20 to 100 percent.

Experiments with the use of royal jelly on humans have also been conducted. Briefly, scientific experience has shown that preparations containing royal jelly are helpful for preventing or treating vascular diseases, especially hardening of the arteries and various other conditions associated with the aging process.

Constituents In Royal Jelly. Researchers have analyzed royal jelly and found that it contains protein, several types of natural sugars, unsaturated fats, a number of enzymes, and is tremendously rich in pantothenic acid, nucleic acid, and vitamin B_6. When animals were given only one of the last three nutrients in larger than normal amounts, their life span increased by approximately one-third. When generous quantities of all three nutrients were given, their life span increased by nearly half. Pantothenic acid has been found to relieve painful burning feet and the pain of neuritis. Some people have reported increased energy and considerable memory improvement after taking this important nutrient.

Reported Uses of Jin Sam Jung

• Mrs. J.S., a housewife, writes: "Jin Sam Jung has had a wonderful effect on my mother who is 70 years of age. She has more energy and vitality, walks a mile every day, does all her own shopping and housework, and doesn't feel a bit tired."

• Mr. L.V., age 72, was troubled by weakness in the knees, and nervous prostration. Normally an active, independent man, the necessity to rely on others to help steady him when he walked was almost more than he could endure. He was given Jin Sam Jung daily for three months. His family reported that "His symptoms have disappeared, and he is his jolly self again."

• Mr. R.P., a business executive, writes: "I went to the doctor because I was feeling tired all the time and thought I might be anemic or have low blood pressure. After I was given a complete physical the doctor told me there was nothing to worry about, that I was in good health. He said the tiredness was probably due to tension resulting from the family problems I had told him about, and that since the problems were now all settled, my energy should return again in a short time.

"However, as the weeks drifted by, I still felt 'beat.' One day I passed a health food store and became interested in various herbs and herb products that were displayed. I bought two bottles of Jin Sam Jung and took some of the extract faithfully every day. By the time I had finished both bottles I had plenty of energy and felt like a new man."

• Mrs. J.D., a waitress, suffered from painful corns and bunions. She said: "The pain wasn't so bad during the first few hours of my daily work shift but those last two hours were torture. I tried special shoes and used foot baths every night, but still the pain toward the end of each work day persisted. My family constantly urged me to switch to a typing job, but I loved my work and hated the thought of quitting.

"Then about two months ago, a friend of mine gave me an article on Chinese herbs, which I found quite interesting. I decided to try an extract called Jin Sam Jung, and after using it for a few weeks I was delighted to find that my corns and bunions were far less painful, and I no longer dreaded the last two hours of my work day. I continue to take the extract daily since I find it not only keeps the pain reduced to a minimum but also gives me a feeling of more energy and pep."

• A woman in her forties was troubled with irregularity, nervousness, and indigestion. She also complained of broken sleep which left her exhausted. She took one bottle of Jin Sam Jung and claimed good progress. After using three more bottles, she reported a marked change for the better. Her bowels were back to functioning normally and her digestion had improved. She added that she was sleeping well and felt refreshed.

• Mr. A.D. writes: "Jin Sam Jung was recommended to me and I bought some from an herb company. It has helped me immeasurably. My headaches and nervous tension are a thing of the past. It also seems to clear your mind (as well as strengthening your nerves) and allows you to think more clearly. This is important to me since I attend college and need an alert mind and calm nerves, especially during exam time."

KOREAN GINSENG COMPLEX

This is a blend of ginseng root powder and assistant ingredients of royal jelly, PABA, and vitamin E. It is sold by various herbal firms and is carried in health food stores.

PABA

PABA (para amino benzoic acid) is a member of the vitamin B complex. It is often referred to as the anti-gray-hair vitamin, and studies have shown that some of the gray hair of persons given PABA was restored to the original color in 70% of the cases.

Researchers have reported that extreme fatigue, skin rashes, or eczema can result from a deficiency of PABA. It is for this reason that the addition of PABA to the diet often helps to increase energy and to clear up or prevent eczema. And indications are that its use may also help to prevent old age texture of the skin.

Vitamin E

Vitamin E is called the "fertility" vitamin because of the favorable effects it reputedly produces on the organs of reproduction. Studies have shown that it is helpful for building muscle tone and strength and that it is a good tonic to the heart. Studies have also revealed that lack of this vitamin can cause the hair to become dull and fall out and may also result in loss of sexual interest, enlargement of the prostate gland, miscarriages, and sterility.

Reported Uses of Korean Ginseng Complex

• Mrs. C., age 49, a nervous woman, developed a rash on the back of both hands. As a typist and receptionist, the appearance of her hands was important to her and she was fearful the rash would persist. She began taking Korean Ginseng Complex daily and in two weeks reported that the rash was fading. Use of the Korean product was continued and Mrs. C. stated that a short time later the rash completely disappeared. She adds that she was surprised to find that she had also lost her nervousness.

• Mr. A.C., age 60, complained of fatigue and frequent attacks of acute pains across the forehead and down to the eyes. His eyes had been tested, but nothing was found wrong. And no medical treatment had so far given him permanent relief from the attacks of acute pain. Mr. C. said he found that loud talking or wearisome conversations would trigger the pain and leave him extremely exhausted.

He decided to try Korean Ginseng Complex and four weeks later reported that the improvement in his condition was encouraging. He continued using the product, and one month later he said: "I can now engage in lengthy conversations, no matter how wearisome, without the pain commencing. And even if the pain does start, it is only very slight and quickly subsides. And although I still find such conversations somewhat tiring, they no longer leave me so terribly exhausted."

• Mrs. R.T., a middle-aged widow, suffered from headache, fatigue, depression, and periods of sleeplessness. She also complained of twinges of rheumatism during the cold winter seasons. Two months after taking Korean Ginseng Complex she told her friends: "I felt the benefits almost right away. It has meant so much to me to be relieved of the pain, depression, and insomnia. I love my work as a music teacher and now I enjoy it all the time."

CHINESE PROCESSED GINSENG ROOTS COMPOUND

There is a "super" type of compounded ginseng on the market which contains sixteen specially selected roots, consisting of the main principal ginseng root and fifteen assistant and related varieties of ginseng roots. This Chinese processed compound comes in the form of hard, compressed nuggets (shaped somewhat like marshmallows) which are wrapped in cellophane pouches and packed in a box. A tea is made by placing one of the nuggets in a cup and adding boiling water. The nugget quickly dissolves as the tea is stirred. Honey may be added as a sweetener. (This product is also available in capsules.)

Therapeutic and Tonic Action

Chinese processed ginseng roots compound is said to contain all forty-two minerals the body requires. Each of the sixteen roots in the formula was selected for its therapeutic and tonic action on a specific part or parts of the body. For example, the principal ginseng root is for the heart and sex glands; three assistant roots are said to support the bone structure, bone marrow, ligaments, and cartilage; another root is for the stomach and digestion; one is for the eyes; another for the nerves; another to clear up the blood stream; one for the lungs; and so on.

Yin-Fever

Another root contained in the formula is said to prevent or effectively treat "Yin-Fever." In this condition there is no fever involved. As one Chinese herbalist explained:

"There are many people who have aches and pains, and their bodies grow weaker and weaker, but they have no fever. This condition is known to the Chinese herbalists as Yin-Fever. Sometimes a person will get what is called a 'spur' underneath the leg. That's Yin-Fever in the bone.

"People who have this ailment do not know what is wrong with them, and their medical doctors cannot find the trouble either. No Western doctor can detect Yin-Fever, only the Chinese can do so."

Special Directions

Vitamin C or acidy fruits or fruit juices should be avoided for three hours after you take the Chinese processed ginseng roots compound. The Chinese also say that it is best to drink the tea hot, and if the capsules are used they should be swallowed with a glass of hot water.

Reported Uses

• Miss T., age 52, was saddled with much responsibility. In addition to her busy career she had to deal with home affairs and an elderly brother who relied on her completely. For some years she suffered from general tiredness, eye strain, indigestion, and nervous headache.

After drinking Chinese Processed Ginseng Roots Compound Tea for a few weeks, she said: "The indigestion, headaches, and eye strain have noticeably improved, and I'm no longer so terribly tired." Use of the tea was continued for some time, after which Miss T. reported: "All my symptoms have disappeared, and I have the energy and vitality to perform all my many duties quite satisfactorily."

• Mr. F. gives the following account:

"I had been going to a medical specialist for several months for a nasty sinus and throat inflammation and had been coughing for about a year. A neighbor who believes in health foods and natural remedies gave me a half box of Chinese Processed Ginseng Roots Compound Tea which she had on hand. Within two weeks of my using it there was a definite improvement. The coughing and throat inflammation had greatly subsided. However, by this time I had run out of the tea, so about two weeks later the coughing and the inflammation started up again. Since the tea is the only thing that has helped my condition, I have ordered a large supply and plan to use it daily because I believe it will eventually cure me."

• Mrs. J.G., age 45:

"Some of our relatives suggested that my husband and I try Chinese Processed Ginseng Roots Compound Tea to see if we received the same benefits they had obtained. We did indeed. We found it gave us more vitality, energy, and an all-around feeling of good health."

• Mr. R.V.:

"I had a very good result with the use of Chinese Processed Ginseng Roots Compound Tea. For two years I suffered off and on from poor appetite and acid stomach. I could hardly eat anything because of the burning acid pain I would have after. The relief from the acid condition and the pick-up in appetite I felt after using the tea were remarkable."

• Mr. J.S. writes:

"My wife suffered aches and pains and was terribly tired all the time, but three different medical doctors could find nothing wrong. She took aspirin to relieve the pain, but the relief was only temporary.

"As the weeks passed, I became alarmed because she seemed to be growing weaker. Someone told me that Chinese ginseng was a strengthener so I went to a health food store to buy some. There was a number of different ginseng products on the shelf, and after looking them over I decided on the Chinese Processed Ginseng Roots Compound Tea and bought six boxes. After she used the first box, my wife's strength started to improve, and we were both astonished that her aches and pains were lessening. Her improvement continued as she kept drinking the tea faithfully every day. By the time the remaining boxes were finished, she had become so healthy and completely pain-free that we could hardly believe it. We are both very happy."

• Mrs. G.H.:

"I don't know if Ginseng Roots Compound Tea would help everyone who has asthma, but in my case it did wonders. I suffered from a very bad case of asthma and had to go to the doctor all the time. I tried Chinese Processed Ginseng Roots Compound Tea and it helped, so I began taking it all the time and still do. I haven't had to go to the doctor for over six months now because I've not had any more asthmatic attacks since drinking the Chinese tea."

• An Oriental man, 76 years of age, stated that the nugget form of Ginseng Roots Compound helped him to recover from a long-standing illness. He reported that even after he was well, he continued drinking the tea as a daily tonic, and in three years his gray hair had turned back to its natural black color.

• Here is another interesting account of the use of Chinese Processed Ginseng Roots Compound Tea. A woman 77 years of age writes:

"I am pretty healthy but have suffered from some hearing loss (nerve) for many years, and it was slowly getting worse. I had never been able to hear the TV when my friend was listening. Her ears were so sensitive that she could not stand it turned up high enough for me.

"I started taking Chinese Processed Ginseng Roots Compound Tea twice a day. Later I accidently broke the plastic tube on my hearing aid. I tried to put on a reserve, but the battery was dead. I was amazed to find I could hear better without the hearing aid than I have for twenty years or more. I still have a little trouble with high sounds, birds, some children's voices, but I do hear some children's or high pitched voices I have not been able to hear for years. I heard the ticking of my car's directional signals for the first time ever without my hearing aid. For the past two weeks, everywhere I go, people notice how much better I hear. I can hardly believe it myself."

• A woman was going through a difficult menopause and had been highly sensitive and nervous ever since her first marriage, when she had suffered three miscarriages. She had been troubled with low blood pressure, an under-active thyroid, a bad back, and severe headaches since childhood.

Her condition was responding favorably to physio-therapy treatments and colonic irrigations, but a recent emotional shock gave her a setback. The patient reported that she began drinking Ginseng Roots Compound Tea every day for some months and as a result became a "new woman."

• Mr. D.S. gives this account: "I suffered from a hemorrhoid condition, nervousness, insomnia, and nasal catarrh. After drinking Ginseng Roots Compound Tea daily, I noted a marked relief from the hemorrhoid condition, a calming and relaxing effect on my nerves, and a noticeable clearing of the nasal catarrh."

• There are many reports which indicate that Chinese Processed Ginseng Roots Compound Tea is an excellent antidote for drunkenness. According to the Chinese, the formula will sober up a drunken person in less than ten minutes and this can be proven by anyone. People who have tried it swear that the Chinese claim is true. When they wish to sober up, some people take two capsules of the Ginseng Compound with a glass of hot water, while others prefer to drink a cup of the instant tea in nugget form. Still others have stated that they simply drop one of the Compound Ginseng nuggets in the last glass of liquor they drink before leaving a party and that it sobers them up in less than ten minutes.

AI-HAO

English Name: Mugwort
Botanical Name: *Artemisia vulgaris*

Mugwort is a species of wormwood which is employed extensively in Chinese medicine. It is classified as a tonic, nervine, antihysterical, depurative, and emmenagogue.

Mugwort tea is prepared by adding one teaspoon of the cut leaves to one cup of boiling water. This is allowed to stand until cold and then strained. Honey may be added for flavoring. As a tonic, the tea is taken cold in small doses, two teaspoonfuls three or four times a day.

CHANG

English Name: Camphor
Botanical Name: *Cinnamomum camphora*

Camphor mixed with motherwort herb is a Chinese remedy given occasionally as a tonic for asthenic conditions when the person is over-exhausted and needs a quick strengthener. For this, a small bowlful of motherwort tea is brewed and then strained, and one-half teaspoon of spirits of camphor is added. Only this one small bowlful is taken. It is not to be taken regularly, but only occasionally as the need arises.

SUMMARY

1. There are a number of Oriental herb blends and compounds sold on the market which bring good results as healing agents or health tonics according to many people who have used them.
2. Oriental herb blends and compounds generally consist of a principal herb or root and several assistant and related herbs or other natural substances.
3. Jin Sam Jung and Korean Ginseng Complex are fortified with valuable nutritional supplements.
4. Chinese Processed Ginseng Roots Compound consists of sixteen top quality roots, each selected for its therapeutic action on a specific part or parts of the body.
5. One of the roots contained in Chinese Processed Ginseng Roots Compound is said to prevent or effectively treat "Yin-Fever," a condition symptomized by aches, pains, and a progressive weakening of the body, but no perceptible fever.
6. Herb tonics such as Ai-Hao and those in which Chang is used can be prepared in the home.
7. As a tonic, Ai-Hao (Mugwort tea) should be used cold and only in very small doses.
8. The Chang recipe is not to be taken regularly, but only occasionally as the need arises.

6

THE CHINESE
"ELIXIR OF LIFE" PLANT

In 1933 *The New York Times* announced the death of Professor Li Chung Yun, a remarkable Oriental whose life span had reached over two and a half centuries! His age (256) was officially recorded by the Chinese government and confirmed by various investigators, including Professor Wu Chung Chich, head of the Chang-Tu University. Li had reportedly outlived 23 wives and was living with his 24th at the time of his death.

An article from the *Golden Age* stated that the antique gentleman gave a course of 28 lectures on longevity at a Chinese university, and at the time he gave this course of three-hour long lectures he was over the age of 200. It was declared that those who saw him claimed he did not appear older than a man of 52.

The *Toronto Globe* carried the following story in 1933:

> Even in the hurrying Occident there will be regret that Li Chung Yun, veteran resident of Kaihsien, in the province of Szechwan, has been called from the scene of his activities, taken off in his prime at the age of 197 years. The cabled story carries no details as to the malady that cut short a useful life, and the inference must be that Li was a war casualty. His marital ventures were numerous, and he, with some eleven generations of descendants, no doubt formed an impressive military unit.
>
> This is but half the story. In the Western world aging men are inclined to boast of their years, slyly adding a few birthdays, but it

94

was different with Li Chung Yun, who appears to have been cheating in the other direction. A professor in the Minkuo University claims to have found records showing that Li was born in 1677, and that on his 150th birthday and 200th birthday he had been congratulated by the Chinese government—as well he might. Men who are old today declare that their great-grandfathers, as boys, knew Li as a grown man.

Dieticians should look into this. It is unlikely that during the first 100 years or so of his life Li Chung Yun knew anything about vitamins or calories; and certainly no radio instructions about setting-up exercises awakened him at the dawn. Early in life—either about 1690, 1750, or thereabouts—this Chinese lad developed a penchant for collecting herbs, a habit that he did not shake off for a century; then he began to sell them. And here is the point: What did Li discover? Some neglected weed that contained the elixir of life? Some concoction which he took before breakfast, instead of the modern glass of—oh, well no matutinal beverage of today will carry a man much past the century mark; so why make comparisons?

Whatever was his secret, Li Chung Yun kept it well. All he let the world know was that it was the part of wisdom to "keep a quiet heart, sit like a tortoise, walk sprightly like a pigeon, and sleep like a dog." But that is merely camouflage. There are people without number today who have the tortoise temperament and whom it is almost impossible to awaken in the morning, but they pass on without any notice in cable dispatches. "Walking sprightly like a pigeon" is among the arts lost by man, and it may be that loss of his favorite herb led to Li's untimely taking off; which is a discouraging conclusion to the life story of a calm Oriental who watched the centuries come and go.

Two of Li's Secret Herbs?

The secret of Professor Li's longevity still remains a mystery. But it is generally believed by various sources that whatever his over-all health program might have been, it included the use of several different herbs, and that two of these herbs have been disclosed. For example, an early article from the *Golden Age* stated: "For two hundred years ginseng root has been a part of his [Professor Li's] diet every day. He advocates an herb diet and disbelieves in any exercise that tires."

The other plant allegedly used by Professor Li, is known as Fo-Ti-Tieng, an herb the Orientals call the "Elixir of Life." (This plant is not to be confused with an herb commonly called Gotu Kola which is known botanically as *Centella asiatica.*) This botanical has reputedly been employed as a tea by the people of the Heung San district of China for centuries.

Some years ago, in reference to Li's use of this herb, Mr. P. de B. Layman, F.R.H.S., M.H.P.A. of the Herbal Research Institute of London, wrote an article in which he said: "Fo-Ti-Tieng is not a plant that would attract attention of ordinary folk, yet it has been renowned among Chinese and Eastern Indian scholars as a food possessing great life-sustaining properties. It was Professor Li Chung Yun, however, whose lectures on Fo-Ti-Tieng and the way to healthy longevity first began to attract the attention of other than native students and introduced the plant to certain European doctors resident in Peking."[1]

Information on the herb Fo-Ti-Tieng and its use by Professor Li Chung Yun was also mentioned in a book by Raymond Bernard, M.A., Ph.D. Dr. Bernard wrote: " . . . It was due to the fact that the famous long-lived Chinese herbalist, Li Chung Yun, who lived to the age of 256 years, used the herb Fo-Ti-Tieng daily that gained its popularity, which led the French government to send a committee of experts to Algeria, where they established an experimental station to study it and led the English government to endow a research foundation in connection with a college in Colombo, Ceylon, for the same purpose. A Hindu sage named Nanddo Narian, when 107 years old, who had used the herb successfully as a preventative of senility claimed that the herb contained an ingredient which tended to prolong the vigor of the brain in old age and to prevent its usual senile degeneration with advancing years."[2]

Studies on Fo-Ti-Tieng

• Dr. Bernard also quoted a personal letter he says he received from an herbalist who conducted researches for over thirty years on the physiological effects of certain herbs, one of which was Fo-Ti-Tieng. An excerpt from this letter is given as follows: "I have been using Fo-Ti-Tieng now for several months, and note it gives a wonderful sense of well-being, especially mental clarity. I gave a talk on natural living recently at a health club and used copious amounts of it a few days prior, and thought it surely made it possible to think clearly . . ."[3]

---

[1]Bernard, Raymond, *Herbal Elixirs of Life,* (Mukulmne Hill, Calif.: Health Research, 1959), p. 20.

[2]*Herbal Elixirs of Life,* p. 20.

[3]*Herbal Elixirs of Life.*

• Professor Menier of the Academie Scientifique near Paris, reportedly analyzed the plant and claimed to have discovered in it an unknown vitamin he described as "youth vitamin X," which appears to have a rejuvenating influence on the brain and endocrine glands.

• Jules Lupine, a French biochemist, also studied the herb and claimed that certain parts of the plant contained a rare tonic property which had an energizing effect on the nerves and brain cells.

• In his article, Mr. de B. Layman wrote: "As a research herbalist, I have given long and close attention to Fo-Ti-Tieng, and have found it in practice to be the finest of all herbal tonics and nutrients. It appears to have no equal in the treatment of general debility and decline. Digestion is strengthened, other foods better absorbed and the process of metabolism increased, with a noticeable improvement in the appearance of the patients."[4]

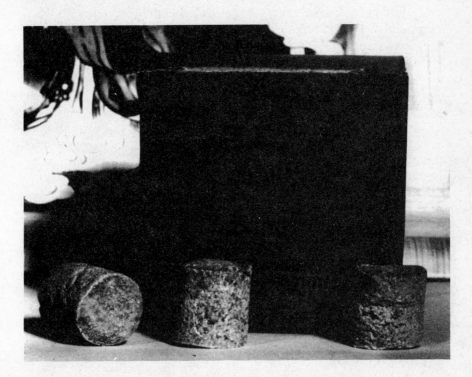

Chinese Instant Fo-Ti-Tieng Roots Tea Nuggets

---

[4] Bernard, *Herbal Elixirs of Life,* p. 21.

Various Forms of Fo-Ti-Tieng

Chinese Fo-Ti-Tieng is available in various forms such as tea tabs, powders, capsules, and so forth.

One particular form known as Chinese Instant Fo-Ti-Tieng Roots Tea is prepared by 28 hours of Chinese processing and is then compressed into small hard pieces about the size of marshmallows. The pieces are individually wrapped in cellophane and packed in cartons. A tea is made by dissolving one of the "nuggets" in a cup of hot water, or it may be dissolved in a cup of hot coffee, soup, or broth.

Many Chinese who have long been familiar with this nugget form of Instant Fo-Ti-Tieng Tea claim that it produces the following benefits: Ten minutes after you drink the tea it is circulating in the twelve functions of the body; it is an excellent tonic, detoxifier, and energy booster; it builds healthy lung tissue; it helps prevent emphysema or relieves emphysema if taken regularly; it is helpful in low blood pressure, but must not be used in conditions of high blood pressure; it relieves the pains of rheumatism, arthritis, neuralgia, and gout; it is helpful for certain forms of eye trouble and kidney and bladder trouble; it shortens the duration of a cold; it relieves certain menopausal symptoms; it quickly clears up hives. In some cases, it reputedly helps lower the blood sugar level in diabetes if used alternately as a "switch-over" with ginseng roots compound tea. (Diabetics should of course check with their physicians.)

Special Instructions

If one wishes to use both Instant Fo-Ti-Tieng Roots Tea and ginseng, they should not be taken together at the same time, but should be separated by three hours. The same rule applies to the herb Dong Quai (covered in a future chapter). If Dong Quai and Instant Fo-Ti-Tieng Roots Tea are both used, Dong Quai should be taken three hours before or after Fo-Ti-Tieng.

Another important rule: If you use vitamin C or consume acidy fruits or acidy fruit juices, they should not be used until three hours after taking any of the above herbs, otherwise the effect of the food value of the herbs would be neutralized.

"Switch-over." The Chinese sometimes use Instant Fo-Ti-Tieng Roots Tea alternately with ginseng in what they call a "switch-over." This may be done in a number of different ways. For example,

Fo-Ti-Tieng is used one day and ginseng the next day, then Fo-Ti-Tieng on the following day, then back to ginseng the day after, and so on, alternating in this manner.

Another example of a "switch-over" method is one in which Fo-Ti-Tieng is used every day for one week, and the next week the switch is made to taking ginseng daily, and the following week the switch is made back to Fo-Ti-Tieng daily, and so forth.

Reported Uses of Chinese Instant Fo-Ti-Tieng Roots Tea

• "I find that Chinese Instant Fo-Ti-Tieng Roots Tea strengthens and clarifies my mind as well as giving added physical awareness and vitality. I use it in the morning before working out. It is a great help.

"In addition to this, I find that it increases what I would call inner awareness. It clarifies and strengthens meditation. I feel it feeds and sensitizes subtle centers of awareness one uses in meditation." —P.C.R.

• "One day a friend of mine, a man of middle age, went to an herb store and asked for Chinese Fo-Ti-Tieng Roots Tea in nugget form. His trouble was that after walking up a flight of stairs he could hardly breathe and was so tired that he couldn't stand it. He went to three or four heart specialists, but no one could help him. After using up four boxes of Fo-Ti-Tieng Roots Tea, he said he is completely recovered and is so happy!"—D.W.

• "I took Fo-Ti-Tieng Roots Tea the first day of the week, and on the rest of the days of the week I took ginseng roots tea. After doing this for several weeks, I have no more asthma."—D.L.B.

• "I am getting along much better since drinking Chinese Fo-Ti-Tieng tea. My arthritis condition does not have pain anymore. Only my finger joints are a little stiff."—Mrs. L.V.

• "My friend and his mother came over for dinner one night, and she had a kidney attack. She had medication at home, but didn't have any with her. My friend didn't know what to do, but since we had some Chinese Fo-Ti-Tieng Roots Tea in the house he decided to give her some. The pain and symptoms left in about 10 to 15 minutes. She has been taking it ever since and hasn't had another attack."—T.B.

• "I had severe muscle pain in the large muscle which runs from the thigh to the knee joint in the back of the leg. Within four days after I took Instant Fo-Ti-Tieng Roots Tea and genseng roots tea, the severe pains have subsided, and I believe that in a few more days the soreness will be gone completely."—S.D.S.

• "My brother suffered rheumatism in the arm and shoulder, plus nervous exhaustion. I gave him three cups of Chinese Fo-Ti-Tieng tea daily, the instant nugget type. About two weeks later he said, 'That Chinese tea of yours sure did the trick. My rheumatism is a lot better, and I have more pep.' "—Mr. L.O.

• "I felt very sluggish and toxic in my body, but the doctors could find nothing wrong. Even my friends noticed that I did not seem to be myself. The whites of my eyes had a sort of grayish look. After using Chinese Fo-Ti-Tieng tea daily for five weeks I feel just wonderful, as though my whole body had a complete inner cleansing. My eyes no longer have that grayish cast. Friends have remarked on my improvement."—Mr. J.C.

• "A friend of mine suffered painful bursitis all over his back. He was also having trouble with his vision being blurred almost to the point of blindness. When orthodox medical treatment did not help, he turned in desperation to a Chinese herbalist and was given Instant Nugget Fo-Ti-Tieng Roots Tea. He drank three cups of the tea every day, and as a result he has no more bursitis pain and his vision has completely cleared up."—D.D.

• "The use of Fo-Ti-Tieng Nugget Roots Tea produced a marvelous cleansing effect in my body. My son also used the tea and cleared up a cold very quickly. In the past, whenever he caught a cold it would hang on for such a long time."—C.J.

• "One summer I indulged in eating a lot of fruit and broke out in a rash (hives). Five minutes after I drank a cup of Chinese Instant Fo-Ti-Tieng Roots Tea the rash vanished."—Mrs. M.B.

• "Since taking the nugget form of Fo-Ti-Tieng tea, my friend, who was weak and constantly complaining of a draggy feeling, can now carry more than 100 lbs. easily. He says he feels so much better in his body, and his energy has increased remarkably."—Mrs. E.V.

• "I was hospitalized for gout. An examination also showed slight traces of arthritis. After being released from the hospital, I took prescribed medicines, one prescription for gout and another for the arthritis, and seemed to be free of these ailments. However, some weeks later I began having twinges of pain in spite of the medicines. I then tried Chinese Instant Fo-Ti-Tieng tea and for some time now have not experienced any further trouble, so I believe the tea has cleared up my conditions."—L.H.

• "My husband became very despondent because for over three years he suffered recurrences of an unsightly boil on his neck, which made him feel embarrassed and self-conscious. The boil would clear up with medical treatment, only to break out again in another spot on his neck in about two or three months.

"A sympathetic friend who was familiar with Chinese herbs suggested my husband try something called instant Fo-Ti-Tieng Roots Tea. At the time, a large boil was again forming on my husband's neck. He bought three boxes of the Chinese tea and drank three cups daily. After using the first box, to his surprise the boil burst and was clean. By the time he finished the remaining boxes there was no trace of the boil.

"That was four years ago, and the boil has never returned. During these years he found that taking just one cup of the tea twice a week has acted as an excellent preventative of any further trouble."—Mrs. J.L.

• "A prolonged and very trying situation occurred and I was overcome with worry and stress. It seems to me that a worrying state of mind can release poisons that devitalize and weaken the whole body, because once the situation had passed, I thought I'd be fine, but instead I felt completely drained and only half alive. I tried Chinese ginseng tea for two months which helped somewhat, but I still didn't feel up to par. I heard about a method of using ginseng one week and using a tea called Chinese Fo-Ti-Tieng the next week, and that one should continue switching the teas this way.

"I followed the program faithfully, and after several weeks I felt just great and had an abundance of energy. It also seemed to make my mind and body function more smoothly and efficiently."—Mr. B.Y.

SUMMARY

1. A Chinese herb known as Fo-Ti-Tieng has been used as a tea by the people of the Heung San district of China for centuries.
2. According to various scientific studies, Fo-Ti-Tieng reportedly contains tonic properties and other valuable nutrients.
3. Fo-Ti-Tieng is available in various forms such as powders, capsules, tea tabs, and so on.
4. One particular form known as Chinese Instant Fo-Ti-Tieng Roots Tea is prepared by 28 hours of Chinese processing, then compressed

into small, hard "nuggets" about the size of marshmallows. A tea is made by dissolving one of the "nuggets" in a cup of hot water, hot coffee, soup, or broth.

5. Many Chinese who have long been familiar with the use of Instant Fo-Ti-Tieng Roots Tea claim that 10 minutes after the tea is taken it is circulating in the twelve functions of the body. Among its many reputed benefits, it is particularly valued as an excellent tonic, detoxifier, and energy booster.

6. If ginseng and instant Fo-Ti-Tieng Roots Tea are used, they should not be taken at the same time, but should be separated by three hours. The same rule applies if both the herbs Dong Quai and Fo-Ti-Tieng are used.

7. If you take vitamin C or consume acidy fruits or acidy fruit juices, they should not be taken until three hours after you take any of the above herbs, otherwise the food value of the herbs would be neutralized.

8. The Chinese sometimes use ginseng and instant Fo-Ti-Tieng Roots Tea alternately, a method which they call a "switch-over." This may be done on a weekly or daily basis, e.g., using ginseng one week and Fo-Ti-Tieng the next week or ginseng one day and Fo-Ti-Tieng the next day, continuing to alternate in this manner.

7

CHINESE HERB REMEDIES FOR RHEUMATISM, ARTHRITIS, AND ASSOCIATED AILMENTS

According to statistics, rheumatism and arthritis are more prevalent than the combined total number of cases of heart disease, cancer, diabetes, and tuberculosis. Other painful conditions such as gout, lumbago, and associated ailments are also quite common.

Definition of Terms

Terms describing the various afflictions may be briefly defined as follows:

When the joints are inflamed, the condition may be called arthritis or rheumatism. If the muscles are involved, the term muscular rheumatism is applied.

When pain extends along the sciatic nerve from hip to toe, the ailment is known as sciatica.

When one or more nerve trunks in other parts of the body become inflamed, the painful condition is described as neuritis.

Pain along the route of a nerve is known as neuralgia.

Lower back pain in the lumbar region is called lumbago.

Gout is a painful affliction caused by excess uric acids in the blood. Attacks occur suddenly and are accompanied by great pain. The big toe is a frequent site.

Inflammation of a bursa is described as bursitis. A bursa is a small soft tissue sac located between parts that move upon one another, often lying between bones and muscles. A favorite site of bursitis is in the shoulder region.

Guideline to Chinese Herb Remedies

Some of the different herb remedies the Chinese employ for the relief of arthritis, rheumatism, gout, and associated conditions are cited in the following list. Along with the use of the herb remedy, Chinese herbalists advise sufferers of rheumatism and arthritis to avoid greasy foods, bread, pork, white sugar, white flour products, and acidy fruits. Meals should include potatoes boiled in their jackets, vegetables, unpolished brown rice, and alkaline fruits. Avocado is especially recommended.

Sufferers of gout are advised to strictly avoid alcoholic beverages, especially beer. Rich foods—such as pies, cakes, and other starchy desserts—are also on the forbidden list.

Those suffering from neuritis are encouraged to include liberal amounts of unpolished brown rice in their diets. This recommendation has a sound scientific basis. Unpolished brown rice contains valuable minerals and vitamins, among which are the major B vitamins, known as the anti-neuritic vitamins. The lack of these essential elements tends to bring on neuritis.

SHANG-LU

English Name: Poke Berries
Botanical Name: *Phytolacca decandra*

This plant grows to the height of about five feet and bears clusters of dark purple berries. According to a 17th century writer, poke root was once used in China as a magical charm.

Poke berries are valued by the Chinese as a remedy for relieving the pains of rheumatism and arthritis. One-half to one teaspoonful of poke berry tincture is taken in a small glass of water two to three times a day. If the fresh berries are used in place of the tincture, three or four berries are eaten before each meal.

Reported Uses of Poke Berry

• "For years I suffered the aches and pains of rheumatism, and I

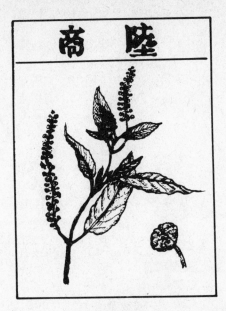

SHANG-LU
(Pokeberry)

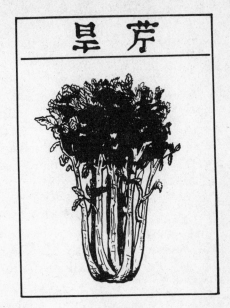

HAN-CH'IN
(Celery)

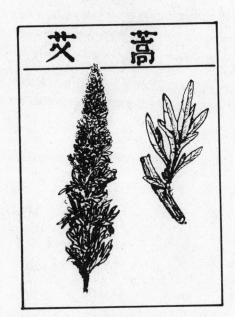

AI-HAO
(Mugwort)

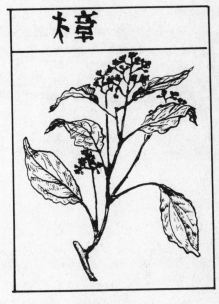

CHANG
(Camphor)

dreaded the damp winter months when the pain would become worse. Aspirin gave me relief, but after a few weeks of taking it, I had to stop because it upset my stomach. I started taking a teaspoon of poke berry tincture in a small glass of water twice a day, and this wonderful remedy completely cured my rheumatism."—Mr. D.F.T.

• "For a long time I suffered from rheumatism in my wrists, hands, and arms, which gradually worsened. I love playing the organ, but had to quit because moving my fingers over the keyboard was very painful.

"One day, during a casual conversation with friends, someone mentioned poke berries as a Chinese remedy for rheumatism. I bought a bottle of the tincture and began taking it. The relief from pain was very prompt so I kept using the remedy every day. Now I can play the organ without the least discomfort. I keep a bottle of the herb tincture in my home at all times, and if I feel a twinge of rheumatism during the winter months, I immediately take some of the tincture, and the pain quickly vanishes."—Mrs. H.S.

• One woman reported that she uses fresh poke berries instead of aspirin to keep her arthritis in check. She says, "I take three or four poke berries with each meal the year around. Keep them in my refrigerator. The weed patch keeps me supplied. Have referred them to many people who are now faithful users."—Miss G.I.

CHINESE INSTANT FO-TI-TIENG ROOTS TEA

Chinese experience has shown that Chinese Instant Fo-Ti-Tieng Roots Tea effectively dissolves toxic build-up in the body and joints. It is therefore regarded as a very good remedy for relieving bursitis, rheumatism, arthritis, gout, and similar painful ailments.

Reported Uses

• "Last night a friend bought some Chinese Instant Fo-Ti-Tieng Roots Tea because she had been having some pains in her arms and back. She took one cup of the tea before she went to bed. She got up and the pains in her arms were gone. She took another cup this morning and afternoon. She called me about 3:30 today to tell me her backache is also gone."—Mrs. G.L.

• "Several months ago I fell and bruised my arm. I took Chinese Instant Fo-Ti-Tieng Roots Tea for twelve days. The results were remarkable. My arm is so much better and I am able to move it again."—N.Z.

• "I suffered for eight years with painful attacks of gout. Although I took the medicine my doctor prescribed and followed the diet faithfully, the attacks did not lessen.

"I heard about Chinese Instant Fo-Ti-Tieng Roots Tea and began drinking the tea daily. I got relief almost at once, and after I used the tea for a few weeks a test showed that the uric acid in my blood had been reduced to the normal level. I have not had a single attack of gout in more than a year now, where before I used to get them about every two months."—B.J.H.

• "Some months ago the fingers of my right hand were so sore and inflamed that I could hardly pick anything up. After I took Chinese Instant Fo-Ti-Tieng Roots Tea for two weeks, the inflammation completely cleared up and has never returned."—Miss J.M.

• A woman 70 years of age suffered for almost twenty years with a bad backache. She said, "I had to wear a brace every day. A friend gave me a box of Chinese Instant Fo-Ti-Tieng Roots Tea, and after one week of drinking the tea I was able to take off the brace because there were no more aches and pains. I still continue to drink the tea every day."

• "I started taking two cups of Chinese Instant Fo-Ti-Tieng Roots Tea per day. In six days I noticed a strengthening in my legs. Rather than having to push up laboriously from a sitting to a standing position, I was able to 'spring' up more quickly and easily. I plan to continue taking the tea."—E.R.

• Since I was given two boxes of Chinese Instant Fo-Ti-Tieng Roots Tea, my rheumatism and general health have improved remarkably. For the first time in three years I am pain-free. So noticeable is the improvement that many people have asked about it."—Mrs. O.A.

• "I had a bad case of bursitis and could not raise my arm to comb my hair without terrible pain. Medical treatment did not help, so I began drinking Chinese Instant Fo-Ti-Tieng Roots Tea that a friend told me about. I took two cups of the tea every day, and in one week the bursitis was gone."—T.C.

• "For five months I suffered wearying rheumatism pain, and all I had been able to do was a small amount of necessary work around the house.

"One day, my neighbor dropped by for a visit, and I offered her a cup of tea, but she refused, saying that just a hot cup of water would be fine. She took something from her purse and dropped it into the cup of water, stirred it a little, and then began drinking it. I asked her what it was, and she said it was an Oriental tea called Chinese Instant Fo-Ti-Tieng Roots Tea, and that she uses it because it helps her rheumatism.

"Well, I thought if the Chinese Instant Tea could help her, it might help me too, so the next morning I bought two boxes. I have been drinking the tea for three weeks now, and it is like a miracle because I don't have even a light twinge of rheumatism anymore!" —A.H.

• "Chinese Instant Fo-Ti-Tieng Roots Tea completely relieved me of a bad attack of neuralgia. I told a relative about the tea since he was suffering from sciatica. He told me later that nothing he used helped him so much as the Chinese tea."—O.T.P.

• "My arthritic hip was very painful, and I just didn't like to be taking drug pain killers all the time. Imagine my astonishment when I began drinking the Chinese Instant Fo-Ti-Tieng Roots Tea, and the nagging pain gradually subsided. As yet the arthritis has not gone, but, oh what a blessed relief from pain!"—A.L.

CHINESE PROCESSED GINSENG ROOTS COMPOUND TEA

Among its many virtues, ginseng is classed as an anti-rheumatic. However, the product known as Chinese Processed Ginseng Roots Compound Tea is said to be more potent and therefore brings faster results than one could get from the use of a single root.

Reported Uses

• A young woman suffered pains in the upper joints of her arms. She said, "All that the doctors could do was give me injections. This had been going on for some months, but the injections didn't cure me. A relative told me she had used Chinese Processed Ginseng Roots Compound Tea with very good results, so I decided to try it too. My condition greatly improved after I took three boxes of the tea, and by the time I finished the fourth box I was completely recovered. I highly recommend this Chinese tea to anyone who has the same trouble I had."—Miss A.W.

• For two years Mrs. G.H. received physio-therapy treatments for pains in the legs and feet. The treatments enabled her to continue her trying work schedule, in which she had to be on her feet all day and work much of the night after she got home. She was able to stand comfortably upon arising in the morning, but her left ankle would begin to pain her as the day wore on. After using Chinese Processed Ginseng Roots Compound Tea for one week, she happily reported that her ankle was entirely free of pain. She adds that she continues to drink the tea daily.

• Mr. C.R. writes: "I know a woman whose friend was crippled with arthritis and believes that the continued use of Chinese Processed Ginseng Roots Compound Tea cured her."

• Mrs. R.D. suggests: "Anyone who has rheumatism should try Chinese Processed Ginseng Roots Compound Tea. I had rheumatism, and the Chinese tea took away the pain, so I don't need to use aspirin anymore."

• Another woman writes: "I had talked to a friend about the trouble I was having with my feet. My feet ached night and day. I had no idea why the pain was there. A friend introduced me to Chinese Processed Ginseng Roots Compound Tea and Chinese Instant Fo-Ti-Tieng Roots Tea. I drank one cup of Fo-Ti-Tieng tea in the morning and three cups of the Chinese Processed Ginseng tea later throughout the day. I had wonderful results in four days. My feet have improved and I am just fine now."

Note: When two different Chinese root teas are used, they should not be taken together at the same time, but should be separated by a few hours, such as cited in the above case.

HAN-CH'IN

English Name: Celery
Botanical Name: *Apium graveolens*

Celery is used in China not only as a food, but also as a remedy for the relief of rheumatism, arthritis, gout, lumbago, neuralgia, and nervousness. The treatment, which consists of a strong tea made from celery seeds plus plenty of celery in the diet, is said to neutralize uric acids and other excess acids in the body. The tea is prepared by placing two heaping tablespoonfuls of the seeds in two quarts of water. The container is covered, and the decoction is allowed to simmer slowly for three hours. It is then strained, and one cup of the tea is taken hot, three or four times daily.

The use of celery as an anti-rheumatic remedy is also well-known to other Oriental peoples. For example, Dr. Kirschner writes:

> Japanese physicians prescribed celery for rheumatism. For one month the patient was placed on a diet of celery in all forms. When the patient got better, people attributed it to the healing power of celery. Since we Americans know of celery's alkaline reaction in the body and of the valuable minerals (particularly sodium) which it contains in abundance, it is not to be wondered at that great benefit was derived from following such a diet.
>
> That most Americans over-indulge in concentrated, acid-forming starches is generally conceded. This results in deposits of insoluble inorganic calcium. Food chemists have demonstrated that the organic sodium in celery helps keep the inorganic calcium in solution so at least some of it can be eliminated. Thus celery helps in both the treatment and prevention of arthritis.[1]

Reported Uses

• "I had been under conventional treatment for arthritis in my fingers for almost a year, and in spite of this there was no progress. The large knuckle of my right index finger was particularly painful and was so swollen I could hardly bend it to touch my palm. I am single and the sole support of my aged mother, so I was fearful that my fingers might eventually become so crippled I'd no longer be able to work.

"A friend who believes in natural health foods told me that the Chinese have many different herb remedies for rheumatism and arthritis. I decided to try the one in which celery is used, so I drank three cups of the tea daily and used plenty of celery with my meals. I also munched on a stalk of fresh celery while watching TV. I did not remove the dark green leaves from the stalks as I was told they are a very beneficial part of the plant.

"Within one month, the soreness in my fingers had lessened considerably, and the fingers were loosening up a little.

"In less than three months, the large swollen knuckle was reduced almost to normal size, and I found I could bend it and almost touch my palm. I have no more pain. There is no doubt in my mind but that a few more weeks on the celery and I will be completely healed."—Miss E.H.

• "For more than a year I suffered painful arthritis and could walk only with a limp. Then several months ago my wife heard about

---

[1]*Nature's Healing Grasses* (Yucaipa, Calif.: H.C. White Publications, 1960).

a remedy using celery for arthritis. She explained it all to me, and also about the diet, so I agreed to give it a try. In addition to giving me two cups of hot celery seed tea daily, my wife also gave me two glasses of fresh celery juice a day, which she made with her juicer.

"I noticed relief from pain in a very short time, and after being on the celery for four months I could walk without a limp. I still drink two cups of celery seed tea every day and will continue to do so."—T.G.

LAN-TS'AO

English Name: Queen of the Meadow
Botanical Name: *Eupatorium purpureum*

This herb has a long-standing reputation as a remedy for lumbago and aching back due to strain or colds. A decoction is prepared from the root and used as a tea.

Mr. G.S. is one of many people who have found the remedy to be very effective. He writes:

"I have used Queen of the Meadow personally and also in one of the most severe cases of lumbago a man could be afflicted with. This man's pains were terrible. I brewed a strong tea of Queen of the Meadow root—about 1 pint of the root to four pints of water, boiled down to two pints—and let him drink a cupful each day, a large mouthful at a time. In less that one week the man went to work."

Compound Formula

A compound formula consisting of Queen of the Meadow and other herbs is said to bring prompt relief from the pains of gout and rheumatism. It may also be used for lumbago.

Lan-ts'ao (Queen of the Meadow) . . . . ¼ oz.
Wu-shih (burdock) . . . . ¼ oz.
Shang-lu (poke berries) . . . . ¼ oz.
Chih-ma (flaxseed) . . . . ¼ oz.

The herb mixture is placed in a container, and one pint of boiling water is added. The container is covered, and the brew is allowed to stand until cold. One cupful of the strained tea is taken hot (reheated) two or three times a day. A small pinch of powdered licorice may be added for flavoring.

EXTERNAL APPLICATIONS FOR THE RELIEF
OF ACHES AND PAINS

TIGER BALM

This is used as a rub for minor pains of rheumatism and muscular aches and pains due to strains or colds.

CAJEPUT OIL

This is a pale green oil distilled from the leaves of the Cajeput tree. It has an agreeable odor somewhat resembling camphor and eucalyptus.

Cajeput oil is used externally for the relief of painful inflamed joints and sprains, and often relieves some of the pain of neuritis.

LU-TS'AO

English Name: Hops
Botanical Name: *Humulus lupulus*

The use of a hop poultice is reputed to bring prompt relief from the pain of neuralgia, sciatica, rheumatism, and lumbago.

The poultice is made by putting a handful of hops in a muslin bag and tying the bag securely, but leaving enough room for the hops to swell. The bag is placed in a container of hot water for a few minutes, then wrung out and applied to the painful area as hot as can be borne without burning. The poultice is covered with a dry towel to retain the heat, and when it begins to cool it is reheated and the poulticing is continued until relief is obtained.

Here is another method that may be used for preparing the poultice. Keep a container of hot water on the stove. Place a colander in the container, but do not let the bottom of the colander touch the water. Put the bag of hops in the colander, and cover the container with a lid. As soon as the hop poultice is sufficiently heated, apply to the painful area according to the previous directions.

AI-HAO

English Name: Mugwort
Botanical Name: *Artemisia vulgaris*

The leaves are steamed and applied as poultices for the relief of aches and pains.

MI-TIEH-HSIANG

English Name: Rosemary
Botanical Name: *Rosmarinus officinalis*

Fragrant rosemary was brought from Rome to China during the reign of Wenti of the Wei dynasty.

Oil of rosemary and oil of juniper mixed together in equal amounts is used as a liniment for the relief of backache, especially lumbago.

HUA-SHEN-YU

English Name: Peanut oil

Peanut oil is used warm as a massaging oil to reduce joint inflammation and pain of arthritis. The joints are massaged three times a day. This remedy works slowly, but is said to bring very good results if continued.

CHANG

English Name: Camphor
Botanical Name: *Cinnamomum camphora*

A small amount of camphor mixed with Chinese wine is used as a liniment for muscular aches and pains.

SUMMARY

1. Chinese experience has shown that various herb remedies can relieve rheumatism, arthritis, lumbago, bursitis, and other painful conditions.
2. Along with the use of a Chinese herb remedy, sufferers of rheumatism, gout, arthritis, and neuritis are advised to follow a special diet.
3. Ginseng is classed as an anti-rheumatic, however the product known as Chinese Processed Ginseng Roots Compound Tea is more potent and therefore brings faster results.
4. The tea known as Chinese Instant Fo-Ti-Tieng Roots Tea reputedly dissolves toxic build-up in the body, which makes it a highly valuable remedy for a number of painful conditions.
5. If both the Processed Ginseng and the Instant Fo-Ti-Tieng teas are used, they should not be taken together at the same time, but should be separated by a few hours.
6. Specific herbs in the form of oils, balms, or poultices may be applied externally for the relief of aches and pains.

8

CHINESE HERB REMEDIES FOR URINARY DISORDERS

Nature's Marvelous Filtering System

Science informs us that each of our two kidneys contains one million microscopic filters consisting of specialized tissue. The blood circulates through the entire body and carries nutrients as well as waste products of our everyday living processes (the collective name for these processes is *metabolism*). When the blood reaches the kidneys, remarkable mechanisms go to work to sort out the various constituents of the fluid. Substances needed by the body—such as water, useful proteins, and so on—are restored to circulation, and the waste products and other unwanted factors—such as surplus nutrients, surplus water—are passed to the central collecting ducts, called the ureters, to be led to the urinary bladder where they are expelled (via the urethra) during urination.

If placed end to end, the capillaries of both kidneys would stretch 35 miles! Each kidney weighs about one-half pound, and these two hardworking organs process between 400 to 500 gallons of blood a day. These figures indicate the magnitude of the task performed by the kidneys. Without this process of purification, the body would continue to accumulate poisonous amounts of harmful substances that would eventually lead to death.

Thus we see that the kidneys are vitally important organs, performing a task necessary to maintaining a healthy life. Sufficient liquid intake (from four to six pints of water and similar fluids a day) plus good hygiene and a well-balanced diet will help ensure good service from the two million filters of the kidneys.

A Word about Kidney and Bladder Stones

Undoubtedly, some of the most painful kidney and bladder troubles are caused by gravel and stones. Excess elements in the system form a nucleus or starting point for gravel and stone formation. Some of the solids, instead of being held in solution and then expelled from the system, deposit in the kidneys or bladder where they gradually accumulate to form gravel. Gravel, sometimes referred to as "sand," is composed of minute particles of kidney stones. Before these deposits of gravel become too large in size, they may be expelled from the body with little pain or discomfort. But when they remain in the kidneys or bladder and continue to accumulate and form stones of a larger size, they cause agonizing pain when they move. For example, the passage of a stone down the ureter from the kidney cuts or tears the delicate lining membrane of the ureter, causing much suffering. When the stones are in the bladder, they are called *vesical calculi*; and when they are in the kidneys, they are called *renal calculi*.

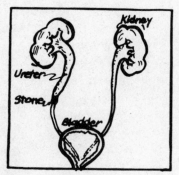

Diagram Showing Stone in Ureter

Kidney and bladder stones are complex disorders involving a number of factors. For example, there are many different types of stones. They may be composed principally of either alkaline constituents or acid substances. Some have calcium as a base, some have uric acid, some have oxalic acid, and so on. Calcium and oxalic acid, both normal substances of the urine, may combine to form urinary calculi.

No doubt you've heard of oxalic acid in relation to certain foods such as chocolate, rhubarb, cocoa, spinach, chard, and beet tops, which are all noted for their high oxalate concentration. If you consume large amounts of such foods without increasing your intake of certain nutrients which help reduce the oxalate concentration, you run the risk of kidney stone formation.

A dietary deficiency of vitamin B_6 and magnesium oxide has been found to result in kidney stones. Other factors also enter the complex picture—heredity, metabolic disorders, and others.

Reduced intake of calcium is usually advised for people who have a tendency to form stones. And according to two Harvard medics, Drs. Prien and Gershoff, 10 mg of vitamin B_6 and two capsules of magnesium oxide (140 mg each capsule) should be taken every day. They report that vitamin B_6 cuts down the amount of oxalates in the urine, and the remaining oxalate that does reach the urine is rendered more soluble by the action of magnesium.

A Word about the Bladder

The bladder is a temporary storage sac for urine which must be voided from time to time. When its elastic walls have been stretched to a certain point, a nerve impulse relays a sensation of the need to urinate. The sphincter, a ringlike muscle which controls the opening and closing of the bodily opening, surrounds the urethra (the tubular structure leading from the bladder to the outside) and is under conscious control. However, very young children often have the problem of enuresis (bed-wetting), because they are unable to control urination during sleep, sometimes due to nervousness, tension, or other causes. Similarly, in the elderly, bladder control may be impaired or the sphincter muscle weakened, and incontinence (involuntary voiding of urine) may result.

Cystitis

Cystitis is an inflamed condition of the bladder and is generally associated with catarrh of the urinary system. Mucous membrane lines the passages to and from the bladder as well as the bladder itself. If the mucous membrane becomes inflamed, it produces excess mucus in the attempt to keep harmful germs and salts from injuring the system. This, together with pus formed as the body tries to destroy the invading germs, may cause the urine to become cloudy and slightly thicker than normal. The condition is symptomized by a dull aching pain in the lower part of the abdomen which increases with pressure when the urine is retained in the bladder for awhile. In very acute cases, pain is also felt towards the small of the back. The desire to urinate frequently is experienced, but the urine is voided with great difficulty and pain, sometimes only in dribbles.

The pain and difficulty in urinating slowly increase, and may eventually become so severe that the patient suffers intense agony each time he tries to pass water, and finally a catheter must be employed. In the condition of cystitis, the urine is generally very acid, whereas normal urine is only slightly so. Retention of urine can also be caused by various disorders other than cystitis. Enlarged prostate gland in the male, for example, can cause difficulty in urinating, often becoming so severe that a catheter must be used.

Physicians mention several possible causes of cystitis, however the main cause is said to be the invasion of the urinary system by the colon bacillus, either directly or through the urethra. Because the female urethra is very short (less than two inches), the condition of cystitis is much more common among women than men. Doctors therefore stress the necessity of cleanliness and strict hygiene at all times, especially after urination and bowel movements.

CHINESE HERB REMEDIES FOR URINARY DISORDERS

In addition to the disorders cited (gravel, stones, cystitis, enuresis, incontinence), there are many other ailments of the urinary system. For example, urethritis (inflammation of the urethra), bladder inflammation or irritability, ureteritis (inflammation of the ureter), nephritis, and so on. (Nephritis is an inflamed condition of the kidneys, and there are many forms of this disease.)

The number of herb remedies the Chinese have for treating urinary disorders are legion. Under the circumstances space will not permit a complete coverage, therefore let us consider a few of the many Chinese formulas and some of the urinary ailments for which they are used.

CHINESE INSTANT FO-TI-TIENG ROOTS TEA

Among its many uses, Chinese Instant Fo-Ti-Tieng Roots Tea is employed for its tonic effects on the bladder. One cup of the tea taken two or three times a day is said to correct involuntary flowing of the urine.

Reported Uses

● Mr. J.R. gives the following account:

"My bladder was very weak, and I had to urinate every half hour. One day my wife met a Chinese-American friend of hers on the street, and she told her friend of my problem. Later when my wife came home she had a box of Chinese Instant Fo-Ti-Tieng Roots Tea which she said her friend recommended for my bladder condition. I drank one cup of the tea and didn't have to go to the bathroom for an hour and a half. I continued drinking the tea, and within two weeks my bladder condition was fine and I no longer have the slightest difficulty in controlling my urine."

● Mrs. V.R. was planning a trip to visit her grandchildren during the Christmas holidays. She writes:

"I suffered from bladder drip, which I found disgusting, and wanted desperately to be cured before visiting my grandchildren. At the suggestion of a friend I tried an herb tea called Chinese Instant Fo-Ti-Tieng Roots Tea, and it corrected the bladder drip very promptly.

"I told my neighbor about the tea. Her husband had to get up several times at night to go to the bathroom because he could not control his urine. After he took the tea for several days, his wife told me he had to get up only twice during the night."

KUEI

English Name: Juniper Berries
Botanical Name: *Juniperus communis*

This evergreen shrub reaches from four to six feet in height and grows on hills, rocky slopes, and edges of woods. It is common to the Northern Provinces of China, but is also found in many other parts of the world.

The berries of the Juniper tree have a pleasant aromatic odor, and scientific analyses have shown they contain a combination of wholesome active properties. In some areas of the Far East and other lands, the berries are used as a balsamic incense. A handful placed on a warm stove fills the home with a lovely fragrance that masks strong, lingering cooking odors. At one time it was believed that burning Juniper berries regularly would purify the air of sick rooms and prevent the spread of infection.

In Chinese medicine the berries are employed for relieving kidney and bladder complaints and for strengthening and imparting tone to the urinary passages. They are also reputed to be helpful in treating conditions of urethritis and cystitis. In addition, the Chinese value the berries as a remedy for other disorders, such as loss of appetite and flatulent indigestion, for which purpose they eat from three to six berries at a time. These berries are said to be agreeable to the weakest stomach. It is also claimed that the distressing back pains of lumbago are quickly relieved by the use of a Juniper berry remedy.

Juniper Berry Formulas

For various urinary conditions the Chinese may use the berries in any one of several different forms. For example, they may use them as a tea prepared from the berries alone, as a combination tea made with the berries and other select herbs, as a Juniper berry wine, or as an oil obtained from the berries (Juniper berry oil).

Simple Tea. One tablespoonful of crushed Juniper berries is placed in a saucepan, and four cups of water are added. The saucepan is covered with a lid, and the tea is brought to a boil and boiled slowly down to two cups. One cup of the strained tea is taken during the day, and a second cup is taken at bedtime.

This simple tea is considered a good kidney remedy.

Juniper Berry Wine. To prepare the wine a large handful of Juniper berries is placed in a gallon of any kind of good quality wine. The bottle is capped and allowed to stand for three weeks. During this period the bottle is shaken thoroughly once a day. At the end of three weeks the berries are strained off and thrown away.

The Juniper wine is used as a kidney and stomach tonic. One small wineglass of the wine is taken a day.

Juniper Berry Oil. Commercial oil of Juniper berries sold on the market is obtained chiefly from the ripe fruit. (Juniper berry oil must not be confused with *Juniper wood oil,* which must never be used internally.)

Medicinally, the oil of Juniper berries is regarded as a powerful remedy for ailing kidneys. In addition to relieving various types of kidney complaints and reducing bladder irritation, the oil reputedly tones up the entire urinary system. It is also said to increase the flow of urine and is therefore helpful as a stimulating diuretic in certain dropsical conditions.

Juniper berry oil reputedly is so active, especially on the kidneys, that it must be used only in very small amounts, from three to eight drops on a little sugar two or three times a day.

Oil of Juniper berries and oil of rosemary mixed together in equal amounts and taken in five to ten drop doses (on a little sugar) three times a day is considered a superb remedy for lumbago.

The mixed oils may also be used externally as a liniment for the relief of lumbago pains.

Combination Herb Tea Formulas

For relieving conditions of cystitis, urethritis, gravel, stones, bladder and kidney inflammation, scalding urine, and various other kidney and bladder complaints, Juniper berries are combined with other select herbs and prepared and used as follows:

One ounce each of Juniper berries, Buchu *(Barosma betulina),* Clivers *(Galium aparine),* Uva-ursi *(Arctostaphylos uva-ursi),* Parsley Piert *(Alchemilla arvensis),* Sage *(Salvia officinalis),* and Marshmallow leaves *(Althaea officinalis)* are pulverized, then thoroughly mixed together and stored in a capped jar. One teaspoonful of the mixture is placed in a cup and boiling water added. The cup is covered with a saucer, and the tea is allowed to steep (stand) for 10 minutes and is then strained. One cup of the tea is taken three times daily (once before each meal). In more stubborn cases one cup is taken every three hours. (If necessary, another supply of the herb mixture may be prepared and stored inside a jar for further use.)

In conditions of cystitis, an accessory treatment is used in addition to drinking the combination herb tea. This consists of fomentations of hot cloths (cloths dipped in hot water and wrung out) applied frequently to the bladder area. The fomentations are continued for a few days. Hot sitz baths taken daily are also recommended.

Note: To give us some indication why the various herbs were selected for the combination tea formula, let us briefly consider the medicinal action attributed to each of the herbs.

(Juniper Berries.) Medicinally, the Juniper berry is classed as a diuretic and carminative. The principal constituent in the Juniper berry is a volatile oil. It is the same aromatic oil that is released when Juniper remedies are prepared that gives the berries their effectiveness and healing qualities. It is also the same fragrant oil that evaporates into the air when the berries are placed on a hot stove.

(**Clivers.**) The medicinal action of Clivers is cited as diuretic, tonic, alterative, and aperient. It is reputed to be a helpful agent in conditions of the bladder and scalding urine.

(**Uva-ursi.**) This contains a glycoside called *arbutin* and owes much of its marked diuretic action to this substance. During its excretion by the kidneys, *arbutin* exercises an antiseptic effect on the urinary mucous membrane. Uva-ursi is therefore considered to be of value in various conditions of the urinary tract such as cystitis, urethritis, and so on. Uva-ursi is also said to be a strengthener of the sphincter muscle, and as such is useful in conditions of "night rising" and incontinence. For this particular purpose, the herb is used alone and prepared as an instant tea, one teaspoonful of the powdered herb to one cup of boiling water. One cup of the tea is taken every morning and evening.

(**Parsley Piert.**) This herb is not related to the common parsley, however its medicinal action is somewhat similar. It is classed as a diuretic and soothing demulcent. In olden times the herb was called "Parsley Breakstone," and to this day the plant has retained its reputation as a helpful remedy for gravel, kidney and bladder stones, and other urinary complaints.

(**Buchu.**) Buchu is cited medicinally as a diuretic and astringent. It is considered one of the best herbs for diseases of the bladder. It is said to normalize the flow of urine, produce a restorative effect on the bladder, relieve irritation, and reduce acid. It is also considered to be a very useful agent in treating conditions of cystitis and gravel.

(**Marshmallow.**) Marshmallow has a mucilaginous and demulcent action which is very soothing to irritable or inflamed urinary organs and passages. Its lubricant properties also reputedly heal the membranes which may have been cut by rough edges of gravel.

(**Sage.**) Sage is regarded as a helpful agent in purifying the kidneys. In pharmaceutical writings sage is listed among the antiseptics.

PIEN-HSU

English Name: Knotgrass
Botanical Name: *Polygonum aviculaire*

Knotgrass is used in Chinese medicine for many different ailments and is especially valued as a helpful remedy for gravel and kidney and bladder stones. The tea is also regarded as a preventative where there is a tendency to develop gravel or stones.

Knotgrass is prepared as a tea. One ounce is added to one pint of boiling water. The container is covered, and the tea is allowed to stand until cold. One cup of the cold tea is taken three or four times a day.

Another Chinese formula consists of mixing one-half ounce each of knotgrass and horsetail grass *(Equisetum)*, prepared and taken the same as the previous recipe.

CHI-TS'AI

English Name: Shepherd's Purse
Botanical Name: *Capsella bursa pastoris*

This herb was given the common name of Shepherd's Purse because its seed pods somewhat resemble an old-fashioned leather purse. It is generally distributed throughout the world and has been used medicinally as an astringent, diuretic, and urinary tonic in Chinese herb practice since earliest times.

A decoction of the herb is employed for soothing and toning up the urinary passages. It is used in conditions of scalding urine, urethral irritation, and catarrh of the bladder and ureters. It reputedly brings prompt relief in cases where mucus is voided with the urine.

The decoction is prepared by adding two ounces of Shepherd's Purse to one and one-half pints of water, and slowly boiling the mixture down to one pint. It is then strained and taken cold, one teacupful four or five times daily until results are obtained.

Combined Formulas

As a stimulant diuretic for conditions of water retention, a mixture of one ounce of Shepherd's Purse and one-half ounce each of Couch Grass *(Triticum repens)* and Knotgrass are placed in a container, and two pints of boiling water are poured on. The container is covered and is allowed to steep (stand) for 30 minutes, then it is strained. One cupful is taken four times daily.

For conditions of mucus or gravelly deposits in the urine a tea is prepared with one quart of boiling water poured over a mixture of one-half ounce each of Shepherd's Purse, Sage, Marshmallow leaves,

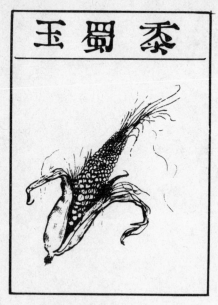

YU-SHU-SHU
(Corn—Showing Corn Silks)

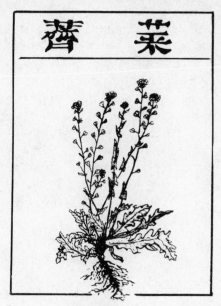

CHI-TS'AI
(Shepherd's Purse)

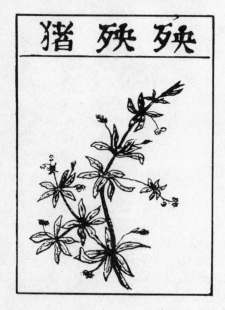

CHU-YANG-YANG
(Clivers)

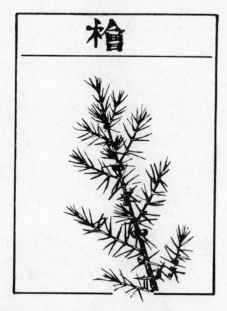

KUEI
(Juniper Berries)

and Peach leaves. The porcelain container is covered, and the tea is allowed to stand for one-half hour and then strained. One teacupful is taken four or five times daily. This remedy is also used for the relief of scalding urine.

INN SAI

English Name: Parsley
Botanical Name: *Apium petroselinum*

Parsley tea reputedly produces a soothing effect on the lining of the urinary passages. It is said to bring great relief to the kidneys and bladder whenever there is irritation, congestion, inflammation, or weakness of these organs. It is also claimed to be helpful in conditions of kidney and bladder calculi.

Chinese claims for the remedial effects of parsley have received some scientific support. Considerable research on the plant was conducted by R.D. Pope, M.D., who reported that parsley is "excellent for the genito-urinary tract, of great assistance in the calculi of the kidneys and bladder, albuminaria, nephritis, and other kidney trouble."[1]

Parsley tea is prepared by placing a fresh bunch of parsley in a saucepan and adding two pints of cold water. This is brought to a boil and simmered not more than 10 seconds. The vessel is then covered, removed from the burner, allowed to stand until cold, and then strained. Four to five cups of the tea are taken daily until results are obtained. (The cold tea may be reheated and taken warm.)

Although the leaves of parsley are the part of the herb most commonly used to prepare the tea, the beverage may be made from the dried roots if one prefers. In this case, a heaping tablespoonful of the dried cut roots are boiled slowly in one quart of water for 15 minutes. The decoction is allowed to stand until cold, strained, and taken in cupful doses four times daily.

Reported Uses

I was incapacitated by what was diagnosed as toxic poisoning accompanied by a tough case of pyelitis [infection of the outlet of the kidney]. For two years I helped support a general practitioner

---

[1]Kirschner, H.E., *Nature's Healing Grasses* (Yucaipa, Calif.: H.C. White Publications, 1960), p. 97.

and a neurologist. At the end of that time I could not walk across the room without help, and I had lost 50 pounds in weight and my pocketbook was a mere shadow of its former self.

During a friendly visit an acquaintance asked me if I had tried parsley tea for the urinary condition. As I had never done this, he gave me these instructions: "Take a fresh bunch of parsley, as obtained in most markets, untie it and wash it in cold water. Place in a dish and cover with scalding hot water. Cover to keep warm. When cold, pour off the liquid, and drink during a twenty-four hour period. Repeat daily until cured."

I've recommended this to many people. They never fail to get a cure, regardless of whether it is a kidney or bladder complaint. I've never known it to require more than three weeks for a cure, and have known several cases where only three days was necessary. My own case required between two and three weeks for a cure, and there has been a lapse of thirty-five years without a recurrence.

A few months ago, I heard that a friend was having kidney trouble. Without further investigation I sent her the above instructions. About a month later I received a two page letter stating that she had been under a doctor's care for six months with two hospital confinements. She received my letter on the day that she returned from the last hospital trip, and was ready to try anything once, and she did. In three days, her urine was perfectly clear, and she was ready to resume her household duties in her mobile home. In a week's time, she was covering the park to catch up on her social obligations and tell the world of her wonderful cure.—H.K.W.[2]

SHU-WEI-TS'AO

English Name: Sage
Botanical Name: *Salvia officinalis*

The botanical name for sage *(Salvia officinalis)* is derived from *salvere,* meaning "to be in good health." This herb is classed medicinally as a natural antiseptic.

A tea made with equal parts of sage and peppermint leaves is said to help purify the kidneys. One pint of boiling water is poured into a vessel containing one-half ounce each of sage and peppermint leaves. The vessel is covered with a lid, and the tea is allowed to stand until cold. One cupful is taken two or three times daily.

----

[2]*Prevention,* Emmaus, Pa., October, 1970, p. 14.

Reported Uses

One woman reports that she suffered from a kidney infection for more than a year. She says:

"My doctor treated me with antibiotics which helped for a while, but the infection returned. I finally had so many treatments with antibiotics that they no longer worked at all.

"Then one night my son brought home an Oriental friend whose father was an herbalist. The young man knew all about Chinese herbs and told me to try a tea of sage and peppermint. The next day I bought the herbs and began drinking the tea. I took two cups a day for three months, and my kidney infection is all gone."

CHIH-MA

English Name: Flaxseed
Botanical Name: *Linum usitatissimum*

The flax herb is extensively cultivated in China for its seeds and oil. Medicinally, a tea made from the seeds is considered valuable for relieving irritation or inflammation of the urinary passages and organs, especially bladder irritability.

The prepared infusion has the consistency of a soothing mucilage. It is made by placing two ounces of the seeds in a container and pouring one quart of boiling water over them. The preparation is covered with a lid, allowed to stand for ten minutes, and then strained. A small pinch of powdered licorice is added. If the tea is too thick for drinking, dilute it with water.

In acute cases, one cup of the tea is taken every two hours; in milder cases, three to four cups of the warm tea are taken daily.

HU-LU-PA

English Name: Fenugreek
Botanical Name: *Trigonella foenum-graecum*

The seeds of the fenugreek plant have been used as a medicine in China since the Tang dynasty. A tea prepared from the seeds is recommended as a soothing demulcent for irritation of the bladder, and it reputedly has helped some people troubled with the condition of "night rising" (getting up too often during the night to urinate).

Fenugreek seed tea is prepared according to the same directions as those given for flaxseed tea, except that the licorice is omitted. Three to four cups of the warm fenugreek tea are taken every day.

HSI-KUA

English Name: Watermelon
Botanical Name: *Citrullus vulgaris*

The common watermelon was introduced into China from Mongolia in the 10th century. Several varieties are grown in the Far East, but the black seeded variety is the most highly favored.

Watermelon seed is classed as a diuretic and considered a good kidney and bladder cleanser for women. Two tablespoons of the seeds are boiled for five minutes in one pint of water. The container is then covered, and the brew is allowed to stand until cold. One teacupful of the strained tea is taken three or four times a day. Watermelon is eaten frequently during the watermelon season.

Reported Uses

Mrs. J.R. writes: "For about 10 years I suffered from a bladder infection. During this time I cooperated fully with my family physician, and we tried many antibiotics, drugs, and sulfas. In spite of this I would suffer a recurring bladder infection about four or five times a year. Then a neighbor told me about watermelon seed tea. Since I felt it was a perfectly harmless remedy and I had nothing to lose even if it didn't help, I gave it a try. What a surprise to find that it worked! I take the tea about three times a week, and I have not had a recurrence of the bladder infection in sixteen months. I also eat plenty of watermelon itself when it's in season and save the seeds for year around use."

Note: The Chinese do not recommend the watermelon remedy for men, as they claim too much melon builds "moisture pressure" in the male body and causes pressure on the prostate gland. (See chapter on men's ailments.)

YU-SHU-SHU

English Name: Corn
Botanical Name: *Zea mays*

Corn as a food crop was introduced into China from the West. When prepared as corn meal it is considered to be a nutritious gruel and an excellent diet for convalescents. Common Chinese names for Indian corn include Pa-lu and Liu-su.

The part of the corn plant used in Chinese medicine consists of the fine silky threads of the stigmas of the flowers of maize (corn). These filaments hang from the point of the husk and are called "corn silk" (known botanically as *Stigmata maidis*). Chinese herbalists cite the medicinal action of corn silk as a diuretic, stimulant, and demulcent.

A tea made with dried corn silks reputedly imparts a soothing effect to the bladder, kidneys, and urinary passages whenever there is irritation or inflammation of these organs. It is said to be helpful in relieving acute and chronic cases of cystitis and bladder irritation caused by phosphatic and uric acid gravel. Another beneficial effect credited to corn silk tea is that of normalizing the flow of urine.

The tea is prepared by placing one heaping teaspoon of finely cut dried corn silks in a cup and adding boiling water. The cup is covered with a saucer, allowed to stand until cool, and then strained. The tea may be taken frequently every day.

A stronger tea may be made as follows: Place two heaping tablespoons of dried corn silks in a porcelain container and pour one pint of boiling water over them. Cover with a lid, allow the tea to stand for one-half hour, then strain.

With either method the tea may be taken in cupful doses frequently every day.

Combined Formula

For conditions of bladder drip, gravel, incontinence, scalding urine, or a burning sensation accompanied by a frequent desire to urinate, one ounce of dried corn silks and one-half ounce each of couch grass *(Triticum repens)* and uva-ursi *(Arctostaphylos uva-ursi)* are mixed together and placed in a porcelain container. One quart of boiling water is poured on the herbs, the container is covered, and the tea is allowed to stand for twenty minutes and then strained. One cupful is taken three or four times daily.

Reported Uses

• Mrs. G.M. is one of many people who has found corn silk to be an effective remedy. She writes:

"Some years back (I am now 83) when I was living in St. Louis there seemed to be something dreadfully wrong with my kidneys. Three doctors, having taken an X-ray which showed the lower half of one kidney completely black, decided that I must have an operation, at least an exploratory one.

"Deciding not to have the operation, I took my family to the country, bag and baggage, and drank corn silk tea instead of water for a year. Upon my return to the city, one of the doctors called upon me and asked, 'How are you?' I answered, 'Just fine! And you are going to laugh when I tell you I have been drinking corn silk tea.' He said, 'Well, that is nothing to laugh at—that is where they get their kidney medicine.' Another X-ray showed an entirely clean kidney. Now I swear by corn silk tea."

Following are three more interesting reports on the use of corn silk tea:

• "My husband broke his hip, and his lying in bed all the time caused his kidneys to become sluggish so he did not urinate as much as he should. A Chinese herbalist suggested he drink corn silk tea, and this fixed him up just fine."—Mrs. R.V.

• "Each summer when we husk our sweet corn we save all the silks and dry them thoroughly. These we place in an airtight jar, and when we need to we take a portion and make a tea of them. This is so good for any kind of kidney trouble. The tea will regulate the amount of urine if there is too much or too little. It can be taken any time since it is absolutely harmless."—Mrs. R.L.C.

• "For several weeks I suffered from scalding urine, bladder drip, and a painful bladder. After trying many things without success, I finally obtained complete relief from a Chinese herb formula, a tea made with a combination of corn silk, uva-ursi, and couch grass. It was remarkable!"—Mr. C.R.

Some Medical Opinions of Corn Silk Tea

Research into medical literature spanning many years shows that the Chinese claim for the effectiveness of corn silk tea has been shared by a number of Western physicians. For example, in the last century *The Medical News* (1881) recommended the use of corn silk tea as a remedy for bladder complaints and the condition of cystitis. In the same year an article by Professor L.W. Benson appeared in the *Therapeutic Gazette,* in which he reported that he found the corn silk tea remedy both gentle and effective. Dr. John Davis, a physician of Cincinnati, reported that a decoction of corn silk combined with dried pods of beans was the most active of all diuretics he had ever employed in his practice.

In later years, Dr. Neiderkorn of Lloyd's cited the following uses of corn silk:

> *Stigmata maidis* [corn silk] is indicated in cystic irritation, due to phosphatic and uric acid concretions. In these cases, the urine is usually scant and of a strong odor. The remedy not only relieves the bladder and urethral irritation, but tends also to prevent the formation of gravel and calculi. It is an important and favorite remedy in the treatment of urinal disorders of the aged, especially where the urine is strong and scant, and throws a heavy sediment. Stigmata should always be thought of in inflammatory kidneys, where it is evident that the inflammatory trouble is due to the presence of concretions."

Dr. S. Clymer adds:

> Where there is a tendency to the formation of gravel, or where it is known to exist, give:
>
> Tincture Stigmata maidis (corn silk) . . . . 1 oz.
> Tincture Triticum repens (couch grass) . . . . . .½ oz.
>
> [The two tinctures are mixed together in a small bottle]
> Dose: 10 to 60 drops of the mixture in a little hot water,
>   as required.
> Dose of Stigmata maidis, in other conditions, is 10 to 60 drops.[3]

The 17th edition of the *U.S. Dispensatory* listed the uses of corn silk as follows:

> Zea (corn silk) has been highly recommended by various surgeons as a mild diuretic, useful in acute and chronic cystitis, and in bladder irritation of uric acid and phosphatic gravel . . . It has been affirmed by M. Landreux to be a useful diuretic and even cardiac stimulant in the dropsy of heart disease. It has been commonly used in the form of an infusion, two ounces to one pint of boiling water, taken almost *ad libitum* [as much as one wishes]; but the fluid extract, dose one to two fluid drachms [in a little warm water] every two or three hours is an excellent preparation.

---

[3]Clymer, R. Swinburne, *The Medicines of Nature* (Quakertown, Pennsylvania: The Humanitarian Society Reg., 1960), p. 111.

CH'IAO-MAI

English Name: Buckwheat
Botanical Name: *Fagopyrum esculentum*

Buckwheat honey is among the various Chinese remedies used for bedwetting. From one teaspoonful to a tablespoonful of buckwheat honey, taken at bedtime, has proved effective in many cases. Consider the following examples:

• "My seven-year-old son was a bedwetter until he was given a tablespoonful of buckwheat honey at bedtime."—Mrs. F.H.

• "A teaspoonful of buckwheat honey, taken at bedtime, cured our neighbor's four-year-old daughter of bedwetting. Some of our relatives have children who wet the bed, so we told them about the honey remedy. It has worked wonders for all these children."—Mrs. L.T.

• "Our ten-year-old son was a bedwetter. We tried everything we could think of to help, but nothing worked. Because of his problem he could not go to summer camp with the other boys, nor could he accept invitations to stay overnight at his friend's house. We became very concerned since we could see that his bedwetting condition was gradually affecting his personality, causing him to become shy and withdrawn.

"Then someone at my husband's office told him about a Chinese remedy of using buckwheat honey for bedwetting. We gave our son a tablespoonful of honey that night, and it was like a miracle to find the bed dry in the morning. We have given him the honey every night for three months, and he has never wet the bed in all that time."—Mrs. J.B.

MUI

English Name: Cranberry
Botanical Name: *Vaccinitium macrocarpon*

Our common cranberry is called "Mui" by the Chinese because it resembles a small plum or tiny peach in shape. Drinking the freshly expressed juice of ripe cranberries is regarded as a helpful remedy for relieving some types of infections of the kidneys, bladder, and urinary tract. It is also employed in some cases of bedwetting.

If fresh cranberries are unavailable, bottled commercial cranberry juice is used. Four to six ounces of the juice are taken three times a day for kidney, bladder, and urinary infections. This is repeated daily for at least two or three weeks, or longer if necessary, until results are obtained.

In conditions of bedwetting, four ounces of the juice is taken once a day, around three or four o'clock in the afternoon.

Reported Uses

• "My twelve-year-old son wet the bed every night for as long as I can remember. I heard that Chinese herbalists sometimes recommended cranberry juice for bedwetting, so I gave him four ounces every day, and it completely stopped his bedwetting."—Mrs. D.G.

• "For eight months I suffered a bladder infection and visited two different urologists. In spite of their treatments, the infection persisted. My daughter suggested I try a Chinese herbalist since these people seemed to have much healing wisdom. The herbalist told me to drink a glass of cranberry juice three times a day for two or three weeks, and I followed his instructions to the letter. At the end of two weeks I had my bladder tested by a urologist, and the infection was gone."—Mr. C.S.

• "Our teenage son wet the bed twice a night for the past two years. He had a kidney infection and passed cloudy, discolored water. A small fortune was spent on medical treatments with little relief, so our family doctor finally advised that we take the boy to a specialist. Before the date of the appointment with the specialist, a friend told me that cranberry juice had cleared up her daughter's urinary infection and bedwetting problem.

"I bought a bottle of cranberry juice and gave my son four ounces about mid-afternoon. That night he didn't wet the bed. He has taken the juice daily for a year now and has slept dry every night except once. His kidney infection cleared up after he was on the juice for three weeks. The appointment with the specialist was never kept. Our family doctor checked my son and gave him a clean bill of health."—Mrs. C.T.

Science Evaluates Cranberry Juice

According to an article in *The Times Record,* Dr. George B. Ceresia of the Albany College of Pharmacy reported that of sixty adults with definite symptoms of urinary tract infection, all received beneficial results when treated with 16 ounces of commercial cranberry juice daily for a period of three weeks. Twenty-two of the patients were considered cured in that the bacteria count was sharply reduced, while others obtained varying degrees of improvement. Dr. Ceresia's experiments also showed that the juice of cranberries aids in the effectiveness of drugs used to relieve urinary disorders.

CHINESE SUPER OLD FASHIONED COMPOUND HERB TEA

This is an ancient Chinese formula consisting of several herbs processed, compounded, and prepared as a tea by a traditional method unknown to the outside world. For thousands of years the Chinese people of the Heung San district in China have used this compound herb tea for relieving or preventing various ailments of the urinary system, such as inflammatory disorders of the kidneys and bladder, kidney obstructions by albuminous conditions, certain diseases of the urethra and ureter, and so on. Reputedly the tea also dissolves or removes those small, excruciatingly painful kidney stones and gravel which so many people tend to develop. But that is not all, many Chinese men have long used this ancient herb compound, claiming that it prevents or relieves prostate trouble (see chapter on men's ailments).

Chinese Super Old Fashioned Compound Herb Tea comes already prepared in liquid form packed in jars. There are three strengths. The regular one is called "Fancy"; the stronger ones are called Super 1 and Super 2.

How the "Fancy" Herb Compound Is Used

According to the Chinese, the "Fancy" herb compound produces a cleansing and healing effect on the urinary organs and passages. It is simple to use. The tea contained in the jar is poured into a porcelain or enamel pot, the pot is covered with a lid, and the tea is heated until it is warm enough to drink. It is taken on an empty stomach.

One jar of the Fancy Chinese tea is taken once every day until the ailment has cleared up, then one jar may be taken once a month or every other month thereafter as a preventative measure against any recurrence of the problem.

Many Chinese people who have never been troubled by any type of urinary ailments drink one jar of the Fancy compound tea a month, claiming that it acts as an effective preventative against ever getting such disorders.

Super 1 and Super 2

For more stubborn urinary problems, the Chinese use the stronger strengths of the compound tea. The treatment requires a set of two jars of tea, one large and one small, called respectively, Chinese Super 1 Old Fashioned Compound Herb Tea and Chinese Super 2 Old Fashioned Compound Herb Tea.

The tea of the Super 1 jar is emptied into an enamel or porcelain pot, covered with a lid, heated until warm enough to drink, and taken on an empty stomach. *Three hours* after you drink the Super 1 tea, the Super 2 compound tea is heated in the same way and immediately taken warm on an empty stomach. The Chinese stress the importance of these directions, stating that it is a "must" to drink the Super 2 tea *three hours* after drinking the Super 1 tea if results are to be obtained.

It is said that quite often just one treatment consisting of the Super 1 and Super 2 compound teas is sufficient to bring about excellent results. However, if the condition does not completely respond to one treatment, the two teas may be taken again the following day, or if necessary for a few days, until the desired results are fully achieved.

According to the Chinese, centuries of experience have proven that the Old Fashioned Fancy and the Super 1 and Super 2 Compound Herb teas are absolutely harmless.

Further Directions

When heating any of these teas, care must be taken that the steamy droplets that form on the inside lid of the pot are not allowed to drop into the tea since this would cause the brew to lose a little of its strength.

The Chinese also instruct that for best results when you use either the Fancy Compound Tea or the Super 1 and Super 2 set, no fruits or vegetables should be eaten for 48 hours after drinking the tea(s). They explain that the omission of fruits and vegetables from the diet during this 48 hour period allows the herb tea to remain longer in the body, thereby giving it more time to produce its beneficial effects.

Reported Uses

• The manager of a print shop stated that his wife suffered from bladder pain and difficulty in urinating. She had undergone medical treatment for some time, but without results. After she took three bottles of the Fancy Old Fashioned Chinese Herb Compound Tea (one a day for three days) her condition completely cleared up.

• The following letter was written by a reflex therapist:

"There is a Chinese herb formula known as Chinese Super Old Fashioned Compound Herb Tea which seems to have a particular value. I personally know of several people who were troubled with gravel and with stones (kidney, gallbladder, and so on), and they have had almost immediate relief after using the Chinese herb compound, with no recurrence of pain or distress. One man was in pain daily and had relief the day he took one set of Super 1 and Super 2 jars of tea. Several months later he said he had no further trouble.

"One interesting thing about this Old Fashioned Chinese Herb Compound is that it does not have to be used for a long period of time to get results. In every case I know of it has only taken one or two applications of the Super herb compound, set 1 and 2, to get results.

"I've never known of any Chinese herb formula for the conditions mentioned that has had such remarkable results so consistantly with so many people."

• Mrs. R.V. writes:

"My trouble began with a dull, aching pain in the bladder and a feeling of needing to urinate frequently though the urine was voided in only very small amounts. The difficulty and pain continually worsened until I had to strain terribly to pass even a few dribbles of water. I became very weakened and prostrated from the prolonged effort and straining to pass water, and my bladder remained so full that I became alarmed.

"I went to a doctor and he diagnosed my condition as cystitis. He inserted a catheter, and I experienced profound relief as the urine was drawn from my bladder. The doctor left the catheter in and strapped a bag to the upper thigh of my leg so the urine could flow freely into the bag both day and night. Of course, I had to empty the bag as necessary. In addition, I was given antibiotics and other medication.

"After one month the catheter and bag were removed, but the prescriptions were continued. Once the catheter was removed I found I could eliminate a good amount of urine without the least strain. However, I had to continue seeing the doctor twice a week to be catheterized since he said I was still not able to completely empty my bladder by myself, that a certain amount of urine always remained in the bladder.

"I continued the treatment for a full year and grew weary of going to the doctor so often for such a long time, and the medical expenses were causing a financial hardship for me.

"Then one day a friend suggested I try a Chinese formula called Super Old Fashioned Compound Herb Tea. She explained that her brother had suffered from a problem similar to mine and had been greatly helped by the herb tea.

"I bought four jars called the Super 1 and Super 2 and drank the first two jars according to directions. In a few hours I got results, and I found I could urinate more completely than I had been able to do in a year. The following day I took the second two jars of the tea. When I went back to my doctor on my next appointment he was very pleased to find I was able to completely empty my bladder, so there was no need to use the catheter. My doctor kept a close check on me for several weeks, and never once in all that time did he need to use the catheter, so he finally dismissed me as cured.

"It has been nine months since I took the four jars of the Super Old Fashioned Chinese Herb teas, and I have taken one jar of the Fancy once every other month since and have never had a recurrence of my urinary problems."

• One man suffered from painful gravel. He reported that he drank one bottle of the Fancy Chinese Old Fashioned Herb Tea every day for eight days and urinated a lot of "dirty, gritty water." He drank the tea for two more days and stated that his urine was perfectly clear and that he felt fine again.

• In another case, a man reported that drinking a jar of the Fancy herb compound tea once a day for six days dissolved a small kidney and bladder stone.

• One woman wrote: "Some time ago I had painful, scalding urine. God Himself knows how I suffered! I had pills from the drug store and medicine from the doctor, but nothing helped. Then I read somewhere that the Chinese people use an ancient herb remedy called Old Fashioned Super Compound Herb Tea for scalding urine and other urinary troubles.

"I bought three bottles of the kind called 'Fancy' and got immediate, blessed relief after taking only one bottle. I finished the two remaining bottles in the next two days and have not had a return of the miserable scalding urine in over a year now."

• Mr. I.L. writes:

"I had kidney trouble and kidney pains for about a year. My urine was a greyish, cloudy color with gritty deposits, and this condition persisted in spite of costly medical treatment.

"Three months ago I heard with interest about the favorable effects of Chinese Super Old Fashioned Herb Compound Tea on the kidneys and bladder. After drinking one jar of the Fancy type of the herb tea once every day for a little more than a week, my urine appeared crystal clear, and there has been no pain in the kidney since."

• Mr. C.C. gives the following account:

"About two years ago I began to suffer pain in the bladder which slowly became worse as the days passed. After three weeks the pain had increased considerably, and other symptoms began to appear, which consisted of kidney pain and intense pain in the left ureter. I visited several different physicians, and each one diagnosed my problem as inflammation of the three organs, but none of them were able to relieve the condition.

"The pains tormented me constantly so that I could not get through a day without pain killers nor sleep without sleeping pills. Then, fortunately, my attention was called to a remedy named Chinese Super Old Fashioned Compound Herb Tea.

"I bought four sets of the Super 1 and Super 2 compound tea and immediately began treatment according to the directions. Results were not long in coming. The first day, large amounts of albuminous matter and uric acid crystals were voided with the urine, and this brought a marked decrease in the bladder, kidney, and ureter pains.

"I continued the treatment daily for the next three days and was astonished at the masses of uric acid crystals that were being continually excreted. After I took the last two bottles of the tea, my urine became absolutely clear, and I was entirely free of all my sufferings. I have remained free of this terrible condition for more than two years now since I take one bottle of the 'Fancy' Chinese Old Fashioned Herb Tea every four weeks faithfully, as a preventative."

SUMMARY

1. The two kidneys are Nature's marvelous filtering system, performing a task essential to maintaining a healthy life.
2. Sufficient liquid intake, plus good hygiene and proper diet, helps ensure good service from the two million filters of the kidneys.
3. Some of the solids, instead of being held in solution and then expelled from the system, deposit in the kidneys or bladder where they gradually accumulate to form gravel or stones.
4. Kidney and bladder stones are complex disorders involving a number of factors.
5. When stones are in the kidney they are called renal calculi; when they are in the bladder, they are called vesical calculi.
6. Cystitis is an inflamed condition of the urinary bladder, accompanied by pain and difficulty in urinating, often becoming so severe that a catheter must be employed to withdraw the urine.
7. In addition to disorders such as cystitis, gravel, or stones, there are many other ailments that can affect the urinary system.
8. The Chinese have a great variety of herb remedies for coping with various urinary problems.
9. Chinese Super Old Fashioned Compound Herb Tea is an ancient formula that comes in different strengths: the regular strength called "Fancy" and the stronger strengths called Super 1 and Super 2.
10. Chinese Old Fashioned Compound Herb teas are taken on an empty stomach. Fruits and vegetables should be avoided for 48 hours after drinking the tea(s).
11. If you use the Super 1 and Super 2 set of Chinese Old Fashioned Compound Herb Tea, it is important that the Super 2 be taken three hours after you drink the Super 1.
12. When you heat the Chinese Old Fashioned Compound Herb tea(s), care should be taken when removing the cover of the container so that the steamy droplets that form on the inside of the lid do not fall into the tea since this would cause the brew to lose a little of its strength.

9

CHINESE HERB REMEDIES FOR MEN'S AILMENTS

The Prostate Gland

According to scientific estimates, some difficulty with the prostate gland affects almost every American man over the age of fifty. Some medical authorities place the age even lower. For example, referring to the estimates of many physicians, Robert M. Overton, a leading chiropractor, wrote: "For many years the medics have propounded the fact that all men over forty should expect prostate trouble. It appears they are correct." (Because prostate trouble is a rather common occurrence in men as they grow older, it does not mean that younger men are immune to the problem.)

Although most males of adult age have heard of prostate trouble, and many suffer from it, few really know much of anything about it. Under the circumstances, it would be helpful to acquaint ourselves with at least a few basic facts regarding the important prostate gland and the various ailments that can affect it. Without going into lengthy, minute details and technicalities, the following information should suffice.

The prostate gland is situated at the neck of the bladder and is normally about the size of a chestnut. This gland plays some part in the reproduction of the species and is said to add a thin alkaline secretion to the seminal fluid. The urine exits from the bladder and empties through the long narrow tube called the urethra, which carries the urine out through the penis in a man. It is the same urethra through which seminal fluid is ejaculated during sexual intercourse. Since the sex glands must empty their secretions into the narrow tube, it is obvious that the urethra must be intimately connected with these glands. This is the reason why a disorder or malfunction of the prostate (which is a sex gland) is most frequently connected with urination.

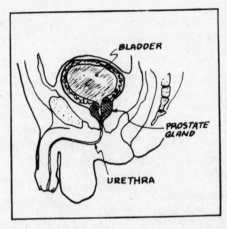

Position of Prostate Gland, Urethra, and Bladder

Enlarged Prostate

When the prostate gland enlarges, it presses against the neck of the bladder which it surrounds, constricting the urethra and preventing the bladder from completely emptying itself. According to medical authorities, one of the earliest signs of a swollen prostate is difficulty in urinating. The stream of urine may become weak and not as forceful as it normally should be. You may experience a sense of not completely emptying your bladder. The residual urine, that is, the urine remaining trapped in the bladder, causes the bladder to fill up more quickly than before, and you find that frequent voiding during the day and the night becomes necessary.

If the condition is not treated, infection usually occurs, causing throbbing pain and sometimes mucus discharges.

Because of its anatomical position circling the urethra, if the prostate continues to enlarge, a complete stoppage of urine results, which is known as stricture. This condition is extremely painful and can often only be relieved by insertion of a catheter (a rubber or plastic tube) into the urethra for withdrawal of the urine from the bladder. It should be pointed out, however, that retention of urine may be caused by disorders other than enlarged prostate. Cystitis, for example, can cause difficulty in urinating, often becoming so severe that a catheter must be used. (If the serious condition of complete urine stoppage is not treated, it can be fatal.)

Prostate Infection

Symptoms of prostate infection generally include backache, extreme impairment of sexual potency, burning on urination, and sometimes a slight discharge.

John Eichenlaub, M.D. gives directions for a home-test in determining whether the condition is prostate infection or urethritis (inflammation of the urethra). He writes: "One helpful home-test is the three-glass procedure. Pass a few drops of urine in one glass, almost all of what remains in another glass, and the last teaspoonful in a third. Cloudiness in the first glass only usually points to urethritis, while cloudiness in both the first and third glasses almost always means prostate infection."[1]

Prostatitis

Inflammation of the prostate gland is called *prostatitis*. The condition may be symptomized by infection and/or pain in the bladder region, frequency of urination, blood in the urine, and so on. Dr. Ask-Upmark of Sweden describes prostatitis as it occurs both in "acute form and as a chronic disease, in which acute exacerbations [flare up of a condition; relapse of a disease] are highly characteristic. The local symptoms can most simply be described as those of cystitis, i.e. a continued urge to void, and discomfort on urination. Prostatitis has, however, certain typical features. Firstly, the discomfort on urination consists far more of pain than of burning. Secondly, this pain is often referred to the tip of the penis, approximately as in the presence of an advanced vesical calculus (stone). Thirdly, the patient may have a sensation of fullness in the rectum, which can reasonably be ascribed to bulging of the swollen prostate gland into it. This makes the patient try to relieve his discomfort by (unsuccessful) defecation [bowel movement]. These local symptoms are accompanied, in the acute stage, by systemic disturbances in the form of fever . . ."

---

[1] *A Minnesota Doctor's Home Remedies for Common and Uncommon Ailments,* (Prentice-Hall, Inc., Englewood Cliffs, N.J., 1960), p. 162.

CHINESE REMEDIES FOR PROSTATE AND OTHER MALE DISORDERS

Following is a partial list of herb remedies the Chinese use for treating various ailments that can affect members of the male sex.

JENSHEN

English Name: Ginseng
Botanical Name: *Panax schinseng*

Ginseng, the herb prized as a near panacea for varied illnesses, is also highly valued as a treatment for sexual impotence. Its history shows that it was used to pep up fading virility by Chinese men for thousands of years. According to reports that have filtered through from the Far East, men who have passed the spring and summer of their lives take ginseng regularly and are able to satisfy their romantic desires as though they were young again.

Professor Lakhovsky, a Russian biologist residing in Paris, studied the ginseng plant and found that the herb, particularly the wild Manchurian variety, has a beneficial effect on the sexual and other endocrine glands, which increases their hormone-producing activity. He believes that the increase of these various hormones is responsible for the rejuvenating effect claimed by Chinese physicians and accepts these claims as valid.

P.M. Kourenoff, in his book, *Oriental Health Remedies,* writes:

> Asked by the author which of the Chinese-Tibetan remedies he considered best for the treatment of sexual impotence, the late Dr. S.N. Chernych of San Francisco stated, "Ginseng! Oriental healers are successfully curing patients of sexual impotence by the use of ginseng, and sexual impotence is one of the most difficult disorders. I can state from personal experience that the Oriental physicians have cured several men whom I and several other doctors tried to help."
>
> The author can verify this from his own personal observations in the city of Harbin, Manchuria, during the years 1920-1923. Harbin was crowded with civilian refugees and interned units of the Russian National (White) Army. Most of these ex-soldiers had served in the First World War, and later in the Civil War. Nerve-shattered and ill, many of these veterans were suddenly stricken with sexual impotence.
>
> They stormed the offices of regular doctors of medicine, and receiving no help, finally turned to the Chinese healers. It is reported

that all of them were cured by the Chinese practitioners, chiefly with the use of ginseng, occasionally supplemented by, or combined with other substances. Three of six persons known to the author were completely cured by ginseng alone.

When all else has failed to restore sexual vigor, ginseng can be counted on, if there is any hope at all.

Ginseng—a Strengthener of Endocrine Glands

Chinese healers insist that ginseng does not stimulate the sex glands into unnatural activity, but that it is a *restorer* of the normally healthy sexual function that has become "weary."

The power of ginseng as a sex improver has been confirmed by a team of Soviet scientists who have been studying the Oriental herb for a great many years. They have established that the root has a beneficial influence on the sex glands and other endocrine glands, and their findings also show that the effects do not lead to premature exhaustion of the organism, for the herb is definitely not a strong stimulant. Dr. I.I. Brekhman, a member of the Russian team, reports that ginseng "acts only by improving physiological processes. No bad effects are observed after taking it."

How Ginseng Is Used

Ginseng's remedial effect on conditions of sexual impotence is not instantaneous. The Chinese maintain that the herb is not classed as an aphrodisiac in the popular concept, that is, it does not stimulate the sex organ into unnatural activity, but works by rebuilding and restoring healthy functioning. Therefore, men who have used the root regularly over a period of time agree that its strengthening effect on the reproduction system is slow and gradual.

Ginseng is used in various ways. For example, some men drink the tea or chew portions of the root. Others prefer to take it in powdered form contained in gelatine capsules or to use the bulk powder added to soups, broths, or coffee. Still others use it in the form of an elixir or tincture measured by drops or a teaspoonful, while others prefer either a fluid extract or a blend. When the fluid extract or tincture is used, the dose is added to a small glass of water.

Some men prefer the super type of Compounded Ginseng Roots consisting of sixteen roots, which is available in capsules and also in nugget form.

Reported Uses

Following are two of many examples in which ginseng has reportedly proved helpful in conditions of impotence or sexual debility.

• "I am a widower, 60 years of age, and have a young lady friend of 38 years of age who is a very passionate person. I see her twice a week, and it has been very frustrating since I could not perform the male function of intercourse.

"Then I began drinking Chinese Compounded Super Ginseng Roots Tea. I used the nugget type that makes an instant tea when you put a nugget in a cup and add boiling water, and then stir until the nugget melts. I drank two, sometimes three, cups of the tea a day. I also followed the instructions of not eating any citrus fruits or drinking any citrus fruit juices for three hours after drinking each cup of the tea.

"I kept seeing my lady friend twice a week, but nothing happened until one night after I had been drinking the tea daily for six weeks. For the first time in twenty years I felt like a young man of thirty, and my lady friend was extremely astonished and quite excited. Suffice it to say that this was a night of great pleasure. My visits now are always the same as that wonderful night. I keep taking the nugget ginseng tea and wouldn't be without it, but I have been able to cut down on the amount and just drink one cup of the tea daily."—Mr. H.M.

• "My friend's brother was about 35 or 40 years old, and he had recently remarried. The girl he wedded was about 21 or 22 years old. He worked as a milkman and had to get up quite early. By the time evening rolled around he was too tired to be in an amorous mood. After a couple of months of this, his wife had become very unsatisfied. My friend bought a supply of Chinese ginseng, the best quality he could find. It was in powdered form in capsules, and he gave them to his brother to try. After about a month of taking the capsules, his brother said he had obtained wonderful results and was very satisfied. He took one capsule each night at first, but after a couple of weeks he felt that this was too much so he cut it down to about three a week and says it is working very well. He said it saved his marriage."—Mr. D.S.

HU-LU-PA

English Name: Fenugreek
Botanical Name: *Trigonella foenum-graecum*

Fenugreek has been widely cultivated in many countries throughout the world. According to Chinese writings it was introduced into the southern provinces of China from some foreign country and has always been an important and popular ingredient in Oriental curry recipes for lamb and other dishes.

The botanical name *foenum-graecum* means "Greek hay." In the Far Eastern and Mediterranean countries, the herb and seeds were mixed with hay and fed to cattle as an animal sex and general health conditioner. Perhaps the ancients got the idea of including the seeds in their own diets after noticing the improvement in the animals.

Eventually, fenugreek seeds were included in medical botany listings and pharmacopoeias and have been used as a medicine in China since the Tang dynasty. From that time, among the many medicinal uses, fenugreek seeds have been held in high regard by the Chinese as a tonic to the reproductive system, reputedly producing a beneficial effect on the generative (sex) organs. In addition, mild cases of hydrocele are said to sometimes be benefitted by taking the seeds in powdered form. (Hydrocele is a condition in which fluid collects in a sac surrounding the testicle. Surgery may be necessary if the fluid is not absorbed.)

Constituents in Fenugreek Seeds

Fenugreek seeds contain protein and, according to a report in *Biological Abstracts,* "new free amino acids," the building blocks of the human body. Another substance found in the seeds is *trigonelline,* which the *U.S. Pharmacopoeia* describes as the methylbetaine of nicotinic acid—the pellagra preventative factor. (Pellagra is a serious disease resulting from nutritional deficiencies.) The seeds also contain an aromatic oil rich in vitamins A and D and similar in composition to cod liver oil.

The oil in fenugreek seeds could possibly account for their ancient reputation as a sex rejuvenator for the animal or man deficient in vitamins A and D. For the past forty years the damaging effects on the male organs resulting from vitamin A deficiency in the diet have been under scientific study. Experiments on laboratory animals showed marked reduction or complete loss of sperm as a consequence of vitamin A shortage. Scientists in Denmark reported on experiments in which boars were fed a diet low in vitamin A. On this diet the animals' sperm count dropped. Daily injections of vitamin A in dosages varying between 6,000 and 8,000 units gradually restored the sperm count to normal.

Another possible sex-rejuvenating property contained in fenugreek is *trimethylamine.* Scientific studies show that it acts as a sex hormone in frogs, causing them to prepare for mating.

How Fenugreek Seeds Are Used

The Chinese advise that fenugreek seeds be used daily in powdered form, adding the powder to soups, broths, vegetable or fruit juices, or sprinkling it over foods. Fenugreek seeds are also available in tablets which may be used instead of the powder. From eight to ten tablets are taken daily.

The Chinese point out that individual needs should be considered. Some people find the powder works best, while others find they get better results by using the tablets.

INN SAI

English Name: Parsley
Botanical Name: *Apium petroselinum*

The Chinese claim that parsley tea has proved helpful in relieving some cases of prostate pressure. The tea is prepared and used according to the same directions as those given for parsley in the previous chapter on urinary disorders.

The reputation of parsley as a valuable herb for urinary ailments and prostate trouble is not held by the Chinese alone. The use of the tea as a remedy for such disorders is widespread and well known in many parts of the world. For example, Mr. R.B. wrote:

"A year ago I met a doctor who took a trip to the Netherlands. There he discovered what the people use for all urinary tract troubles. Would you believe it? It is the lowly plant called parsley, taken two or three times a day, steeped as a tea, quite strong. The doctor came back and started to recommend it to his patients.

"Ever since I started to take parsley I got relief, both from bladder irritation and prostate pressure. Now, after over a year, I feel so grateful I want to pass the information on to others that suffer as I did."

Another example is that reported by Cyril Scott, popular British author of several books and articles on natural healing. He mentions the use of parsley by a man in his sixties:

"This person was in great distress because he was unable to pass water. The doctor was called in, and a catheter had to be used several times. The doctor told him he was suffering from prostate trouble and would have to undergo an operation. But it was then discovered that he had sugar in his urine, and it would be dangerous to operate while the diabetes condition was present. In consequence, injections of insulin were given. Finally, the patient's osteopath advised him to try parsley tea. The result was astonishing!"

Scott goes on to say that the patient could urinate freely. He adds, "After he first drank the parsley tea, a lot of offensive substance came away in his urine. But the latter soon became normal, and the erstwhile patient is now in fine fettle, and able to play his rounds of golf with enjoyment. There is no more thought of an operation."

CH'E-CH'IEN

English Name: Plantain
Botanical Name: *Plantago major*

Plantain is a familiar perennial "weed" in China and other lands and may be found anywhere along roadsides and meadows. The botanical name is derived from *planta,* a foot, and *ago,* a wort, in allusion to the shape of the broad leaves as they lay on the ground.

Medicinally, plantain has a very ancient reputation in China and is given as a tea for general debility, spermatorrhea, and sexual asthenia (loss of sex power). It is also said to promote fertility.

Among its many constituents, plantain provides a considerable quantity of potassium. According to nutritionalists, this mineral is very important to the health of the body. A lack of it may cause varied conditions such as a weak heart, dropsy, enlarged glands (such as the prostate), upset stomach, or swollen testicles.

As a tea plantain is generally combined with other substances, such as flaxseed (*Linum usitatissimum*), for example. To prepare the formula, one ounce of plantain seeds are boiled in 1½ pints of water down to one pint, then strained. One ounce of flaxseed is placed in a container, and a pint of piping hot water is added. The brew is covered with a lid and allowed to stand for one-half hour, then strained. (If too thick, dilute with a little water).

When ready, the two teas are mixed together in one container and three or four cups are taken daily. The tea may be reheated and taken warm or hot. (Flaxseed contains the valuable vitamin F, a nutrient important to the health of the prostate.)

YEN-MAI

English Name: Oats
Botanical Name: *Avena sativa*

The medicinal action of oats is that of a stimulant, nerve-cell nutrient, and nerve tonic. They are considered valuable as a remedy for strengthening and restoring nerve force to the entire system, with a specific beneficial effect on the generative system. They are used in conditions of spermatorrhea, nervous debility of convalescense, nervous exhaustion, and general neurasthenia. They are rated an effective agent in conditions of impotence or sexual debility due to over-indulgence since they are said to produce a tonic effect on the nerve structure of the sexual organs. They are employed for prostatic irritation.

How Oats Are Used

Fifteen drops of the fluid extract of oats are added to a small glass of water and taken three times a day, between meals. If the extract is taken in hot water, the action is said to be faster; if it is taken in cold water, it reputedly has a more extended influence.

For prostatic irritation or early signs of prostate trouble, oats are prepared as a tea in combination with black willow bark *(Salix nigra)* and celery seeds. One ounce each of oats and black willow bark are placed in a container, and 2½ pints of water are added. This is brought to a boil and simmered slowly for 15 minutes. It is then strained, and the hot tea is poured over one ounce of celery seeds. The container is covered, and the brew is allowed to stand until cold and then strained. One teacupful is taken three or four times daily.

CHINESE SUPER OLD FASHIONED COMPOUND HERB TEA

In the previous chapter we covered this ancient Chinese herb compound and pointed out that in addition to treating urinary disorders, it was also used by the Chinese men for relieving or preventing prostate trouble. For this purpose, general directions for heating and drinking the tea(s) are the same as those already cited in the urinary problems chapter. To briefly recap, the liquid contents of the preparation(s) are poured into a container, which is covered with a lid and heated until the tea is warm enough to drink. When the tea is heated care must be taken in removing the cover of the container so that the steamy droplets that form on the inside of the lid do not fall into the tea because this would cause the brew to lose some of its potency. The tea is taken on an empty stomach. Fruits and vegetables are not eaten for 48 hours after the tea is taken.

Further Directions

For mild or moderate cases of prostate trouble, the Chinese compound formula called *Fancy* is taken once a day until the condition has cleared up, then about once a month or every other month as a preventative. Many Chinese men who do not have a prostate problem (especially men getting on in years) also drink the Fancy Chinese compound tea about once a month or every other month as a preventative.

For more difficult prostate trouble, the stronger two-jar set, called Super 1 and Super 2 compound tea, is used. The Super 1 tea is heated and taken, followed three hours later by the Super 2 tea. Generally one set brings the desired results, but, if necessary, the set can be taken again the next day or for the next few days until definite results are obtained. Once the troublesome condition has been eliminated, the set can be taken once every two or three months as a preventative, or the Fancy compound may be used about once a month or every other month as a preventative.

The Chinese further instruct that whether you do or do not have prostate trouble, melons such as cantaloupes, honey-dew, and so on should be eaten sparingly if at all since these fruits are bad for the prostate gland. For the same reason, highly spiced foods are also to be avoided.

Reported Uses

• Mr. V. writes:

"Three years ago I was hospitalized for prostate trouble accompanied by pain and difficulty in urination. Later the problem returned and I was again faced with hospitalization. This time I decided to try a Chinese herbalist, and he recommended Chinese Super Old Fashioned Compound Herb Tea. He gave me the strong kind, two bottles called Super 1 and Super 2. After drinking the two teas, I got results in ten hours. I have no more pain or trouble urinating. From that time on I have taken one bottle of the Fancy Chinese Old Fashioned Compound Herb Tea every three weeks to avoid any future problem. At the age of sixty I am feeling wonderful."

• The following report comes from Mr. K.W.:

"My daughter sent me crates of cranshaw melons during the melon season. They tasted so good that I could not resist eating them every day. I ignored the teachings of my father in China who used to warn me not to eat too much melon because it builds up what he called "moisture pressure" in the male body.

"I got fever and chills and stoppage of the urine. I went to the doctor for tests and he told me that my prostate gland was swollen and that I must have surgery. He also gave me a tube that I had to insert each time in order to rid myself of urine. I could not go without it. But I didn't want to have surgery, so I went to a Chinese herbalist who was well known for his effective remedies and told him my problem. He showed me an herb compound formula in an ancient Chinese book and said, 'This is the strong one for very bad problems such as the one you have. I will make this up for you.' He called it Chinese Super 1 and Super 2 Old Fashioned Compound Herb Tea and instructed me how to use the preparations.

"After taking his teas, I could urinate without any tube. I kept taking this herb medicine for several days. Now I take it only occasionally as a preventive measure. I have had no further difficulty for more than two years now, but I am also careful not to eat the wrong foods."

• Mr. S.T., 36 years of age, was stricken with prostate trouble and complained of pain in the lower back and side, difficulty in getting the urine started, a sensation of fullness in the rectum, and discomfort on urinating. He said, "Treatment by my doctor gave only temporary relief, and the condition kept coming back every few weeks. Then one day my boss told me that he had suffered a similar problem and said he cleared it up by drinking a special Chinese herb tea. I told him I'd like to give it a try, so the next day he brought me three bottles called Fancy Chinese Old Fashioned Compounded Herb Tea and told me how to use them. After I finished the bottles, my symptoms disappeared, and I have been free of prostate trouble ever since . . . for more than a year."

• Mr. S.K. wrote:

"I suffered from prostate trouble for several months and consulted one of the best urologists I could find. He said my prostate and bladder were inflamed and I also had an infection in the prostate. The medicines he prescribed gave me side effects so I stopped using them.

"I heard from a friend about Chinese Old Fashioned Compounded Herb Tea, so I began using it. A week later I went back to my doctor and he said the bladder and prostate inflammation was gone, but there was still a slight infection left in the prostate. I drank two more bottles of the Chinese Herb Compound Tea and two weeks later kept another appointment with my doctor. Tests showed there was no longer any infection in the prostate, so my doctor discharged me as cured."

• A Chinese-American gentleman writes:

"I took a three week vacation in Mexico and during that time I ate a lot of hot spicy foods. Toward the middle of the third week I became very ill and had complete stoppage of urine. A Mexican physician told me my prostate gland was badly swollen, and, after catheterizing me to get rid of the urine, he gave me a catheter to use until I could get back home to the States and see a urologist.

"I left for home immediately, but instead of seeing a urologist I went to a Chinese herbalist. He gave me two sets of Super 1 and Super 2 Chinese Old Fashioned Compounded Herb Tea, which I drank on two consecutive days. At the end of that short time I could urinate freely without using the catheter tube. These good results were not temporary but lasting. Eighteen months have passed and I am still fine. I take one set of the two teas every two or three months as a preventative."

• Mr. S.L., age 40, gives the following account:

"I began having symptoms of prostate pressure, and the condition was confirmed by my doctor. Since I am a believer in natural remedies, I checked into the herb recipes used by the Chinese for prostate trouble and was impressed by the information relating to a formula called Chinese Old Fashioned Compounded Herb Tea. This comes in three strengths, the regular strength called Fancy, and the stronger strengths called Super 1 and Super 2. Since my prostate condition was not too severe and had only just recently started, I decided to use the Fancy Chinese herb tea.

"After I drank only one bottle my condition improved so remarkably that I considered myself cured. However, since I was assured that the herb compound tea was perfectly harmless, I decided to drink the remaining two bottles I had on the following two days, just in case the prostate needed a little more help. That was over three years ago, and I have never had the slightest symptom of any kind of prostate trouble from that time on. As a preventative measure, I take one bottle of the Fancy tea every six weeks and plan to do so for the rest of my life."

• Mr. J.M., age 50, reports:

"I suffered from prostate trouble and had all the regular, orthodox treatments, but they only gave temporary help. There was a high pus count in my prostatic fluid and urine, and I had to go to the doctor every other week for treatment to keep the pus count down. I also took pills daily to help keep it down.

"There was no relief from my lower back pain, so I tried an osteopath and went to him for several weeks, but the backache persisted.

"Then one day I found out about a Chinese herb remedy for prostate trouble, which is called Chinese Old Fashioned Compounded Herb Tea. I took two bottles of the kind called Super 1 and Super 2. The next day my back pain was gone for the first time in months. Three days later I drank two more bottles of the Chinese teas and found I didn't have to get up nights anymore. That was the only medicine I used, and I had stopped seeing the osteopath. When I went back to my doctor for my usual appointment he was surprised at the improvement in my condition. The pus count had dropped way down. I drank another two bottles of the Chinese tea, and the next time I saw my doctor he gave me a clean bill of health."

• Mr. L.L. writes:

"My prostate drip is cured. I took two jars of the Fancy Chinese Old Fashioned Compounded Herb Tea in two separate weeks. I don't know if the zinc tablets I also took had anything to do with it."

Note: Chemical analyses of the healthy prostate gland and of the spermatozoa (the "male living seed") show very high concentrations of the mineral zinc, whereas the concentration of zinc found in the sick prostate is very low. According to various researchers, one of the causes of prostate trouble could be a deficiency of zinc in the diet. We are informed that zinc is notably absent in the American diet due to refining processes which remove this important mineral. For example, the germ of the wheat contains zinc, but it has been removed from the flour that makes commercial white bread. When we consider all these facts, the comment by Mr. L.L. of using zinc tablets as a dietary supplement is noteworthy.

SUMMARY

1. According to reliable medical estimates, prostate trouble is a rather common occurrence in men as they grow older.
2. Trouble with the prostate can take the form of painful infection, inflammation (prostatitis), or enlargement of the prostate.
3. One of the earliest signs of an ailing prostate is difficulty in urinating. If the prostate continues to enlarge, complete stoppage of urine may result, and the use of a catheter for withdrawal of the urine will be required.
4. Retention of urine may be caused by disorders other than enlarged prostate. Cystitis, for example, can cause difficulty in urinating, often becoming so severe that a catheter must be employed.
5. A simple home-test explained by a medical doctor can help determine whether a condition is prostate infection or urethritis (inflammation of the urethra).
6. Prostatitis can occur in acute form and as a chronic disease. Although the local symptoms are most simply described as those of cystitis, inflammation of the prostate has certain typical features.
7. The Chinese have a number of herb remedies from which to choose for treating various ailments and sexual inadequacies that can effect members of the male sex.
8. The Chinese herbs and herb products cited in this chapter as being helpful in conditions of impotence and sexual debility do not stimulate the organs into unnatural activity, but work by providing the nutrients needed to restore normal, healthy functioning.
9. The ancient formula known as Chinese Super Old Fashioned Compounded Herb Tea is among the most highly prized remedies by Chinese men for treating or preventing prostate trouble.

10

BUILDING FEMALE HEALTH
WITH CHINESE HERBS

There are a number of different ailments—for example, vaginal irritation and discharge, menstrual difficulties, vomiting during pregnancy, and so on—that can affect the human female. In addition, the stress of menopause can leave a woman prone to a swarm of insidious symptoms, such as hot flashes, a kind of rheumatism known as "menopausal arthritis," or that dismal depression popularly called "menopausal melancholia."

The change-of-life also means change in the thyroid gland and the sex glands. Puffiness of the face, a little gain in weight, dry skin, falling hair, and slow pulse can indicate that the thyroid especially is finding it a little rough going. Domestic stress does not help matters, and the woman of the house finds it increasingly difficult to check the tide of irritability, at an age when the children are sufficiently grown to be especially critical. The busy housewife going through the menopause cannot always be sparkling and cheerful.

Oriental Health Wisdom for American Women

Chinese girls are taught early in life about the value of specific herbs for the female body. And they are also taught a few words of warning passed down from generation to generation about the adverse effects of anything cold on the female system.

As one prominent Chinese herbalist explains:

"You will find many American girls in their twenties with arthritis already all through their bodies. I will tell you what the cause of that is—American people don't know how to take care of themselves, especially in the case of women and girls. When they have their monthly period, they eat and drink all kinds of ice cold things, take cold showers, and go swimming and skiing. All of the coldness gets into the body. That's one thing. All right, there's another thing—the American girls wash their hair and go to bed with the head damp or put their hair up in wet curls just at bedtime. Again, the cold goes into their body. They don't start suffering from the effects of this repeated practice until they are older, maybe twenty-five, usually thirty or thirty-five years old.

"And when they have a baby, a few days later they are up running around in the cold, rainy weather. Now, when a woman in China gives birth to a baby she stays inside the house for sixty days, drinks special broths to strengthen her body, eats and drinks everything warm—no cold drinks at all. It is our way of what you Americans call 'preventive medicine.' "

CHINESE HERBS FOR FEMALE DISORDERS

To improve female health the natural way, let us consider some of the Chinese herb remedies that have been developed over the centuries.

DONG QUAI

English Name: No equivalent.
Botanical Name: *Angelica polymorpha*

In different parts of China, according to the variations of dialect, this Oriental plant is either called Dong Quai or Tang Kwei. Botanically the herb is known as *Angelica polymorpha,* but is often mistaken by Westerners as either common angelica *(Angelica archangelica)* or Lovage *(Lisgusticum).*

The root is the part of the Dong Quai plant that is used in Chinese medicine. The roots occur in different shapes and colors, generally whitish-grey or yellowish-grey or, in the case of old roots, an odd dark color. Some roots have only a few rootlets. Others have a fat body with many rootlets, but these are considered to be of poor quality. Some roots are processed and squashed flat like a leaf, while others are sold in bundles like asparagus.

The best quality of Chinese Dong Quai root has a strong pungent aroma and taste, whereas weaker qualities have a faint odor and taste. It is said that Korean Dong Quai is very mild and consequently can be taken more often during the day.

Only the hips of the root, up to the head, are in general use. The upper half is considered a great blood builder; the tails of the roots are employed under the direction of Chinese herbalists for emergency purposes only, to dissolve blood clots resulting from serious accidents and for expelling afterbirth that has failed to appear. A liniment prepared with the tails mixed with other herbs and steeped in Chinese wine is used as an external application for removing the discoloration of black and blue marks.

Boon to Women

Dong Quai root is famed in Chinese medicine for its affinity for the female constitution. It is highly valued as a remedy for building blood, nourishing the female glands, regulating monthly periods, and correcting menopausal symptoms, including hot flashes and spasms of the vagina. It is also used in anemic conditions in mothers after childbirth but is never given to women during pregnancy. Dong Quai has been found to bring relief in a number of cases of menopausal rheumatism. It has also proved very helpful in amenorrhea (stoppage of normal monthly periods, scanty periods) and deficient secretion of uterine mucosa.

How Dong Quai Is Used

Capsules containing Dong Quai in powdered form, prepared only from the hips and head of the roots, are available. The capsules may be swallowed with a glass of warm water or broken open and the contents added to hot soups or broths. Since its taste somewhat resembles that of celery, it adds to, rather than detracts from, the flavor of various food dishes. Chinese herbalists advise that for best results, little or no fruit should be eaten while you take Dong Quai, nor should any other strong root teas, such as ginseng for example, be taken for two or three hours after. Vegetables should be included in the diet; however, since many vegetables are very Yin (weak), a slice of ginger root (Yang) should be cooked with them to restore proper balance.

Compounded Dong Quai

In addition to the regular Dong Quai capsules prepared from the upper parts of a single root, there is a super type of powdered Chinese Dong Quai also available in capsule form which is a processed compound prepared from the upper parts of *several* roots. If the regular Chinese or Korean Dong Quai capsules are used, women generally take two capsules three times a day; if the stronger Chinese Super Compounded type is used, only two capsules are taken daily, one in the morning and one in the evening. In very severe cases, two capsules of the super compounded type may be taken twice or three times daily until the condition improves, at which time the dosage is reduced to one capsule twice a day.

Reported Uses

• "All my adult life I had considered myself very fortunate because I never suffered from any of the menstrual troubles which afflict so many women. I never had cramps, tensions, suppressed periods, or flooding, and so I thought that the menopause would be a cinch! But when it came, contrary to my expectancy it brought severe suffering. All my female organs seemed to be sore and aching. I lost a lot of sleep because just when I was dozing off a painful spasm of the vagina would awaken me, and sometimes this would occur off and on for hours. These symptoms were accompanied by a peculiar anguish of spirit. I had a medical examination, but everything checked out just fine. I was given some tranquilizers, but these only seemed to make the spasms worse and to make me feel even more exhausted and irritable, so I stopped taking them. One of the Chinese women I worked with suggested I consult a Chinese herbalist, so I went to an herbalist in a local Chinatown and was told to take some capsules of the strong Chinese Compounded Dong Quai Roots Powder. The herbalist told me that Chinese women have been taking this compound formula for 3,000 years. Due to the severity of my case he advised me to take two capsules three times a day until my spasms had stopped and my organs were no longer sore and then to keep taking only one capsule twice per day regularly throughout the menopause until it was over. The Dong Quai worked beautifully, and my symptoms were gone within a week. I have found that if I stop the two capsule per day treatment my symptoms start coming back, so I continue faithfully with them and will do so until the change-of-life is a thing of the past."—Mrs. M.L.

• "I am a woman thirty years of age and run my own mail order business. For a long time I had been suffering from chronic female tiredness and low energy. One day I bought a bottle of Chinese Dong Quai capsules in a health food store, and after taking them for a few days I noticed a decided pickup in energy. I could do a whole day's work without fatigue. I take Dong Quai faithfully because I feel it is a valuable food product which supplies some nutrients and vital elements otherwise missing from my diet."—Mrs. J.W.

• "Let me tell you the good which Chinese Dong Quai has done for me. I used to suffer terrible cramps the first day of my monthly period and couldn't be on my feet, but just had to sit around all day with a hot water bottle on my abdomen. Dong Quai capsules completely relieved me of these terrible cramping miseries, and I feel like a normal human being again."—Miss C.G.

• "I took estrogen for three years for my "change of life," but after using Chinese Dong Quai for a few months I no longer needed the estrogen."—Mrs. B.C.

• "Chinese Dong Quai is a superb remedy for retarded menstruation."—Miss L.T.

• "I obtained considerable relief from hot flashes and other menopausal discomfort with the use of Super Compounded Chinese Dong Quai. Every woman should know about this remarkable Chinese herb product."—Mrs. M.M.

• "I am fifty-two years old, and I had hot flashes so often I thought I'd go out of my mind. For the past four months I have used Chinese Compounded Dong Quai, and the results have been marvelous. There are no more hot flashes. You cannot imagine what a relief this has been to me."—Miss T.W.

• "My daughter suffered from menstrual irregularity accompanied by cramps and headaches. Her social life was necessarily restricted during her monthly periods, and this caused her to become very depressed. After taking Chinese Dong Quai capsules, her periods became pain-free, and she is her cheerful, active self again, month in and month out."—Mrs. B.R.

• "I've worked as a hotel switchboard operator for many years. As I started into the change-of-life, I began suffering from menopausal rheumatism in my arms and hands. Aspirin brought only temporary relief, and I feared that if the condition worsened I'd be unable to continue in my job. A Chinese herbalist gave me Compounded Dong Quai capsules and told me to take one in the morning and one at night. Within a few short weeks, the rheumatism pain completely vanished and has not returned in over a year. I still take the capsules daily and wouldn't be without them."—Mrs. J.C.

• "A teen-age girl missed her monthly period for six months. She had been taken to a medical doctor, but her condition did not improve. Her parents were very worried and finally took the girl to a Chinese herbalist who prescribed a bottle of Compounded Dong Quai capsules. A few days later the parents went back to the herbalist and happily reported that their daughter's period had started. They saw him again a year later and informed him that the young girl had never had any further trouble with her periods."—Mrs. L.S.

HSIEN

English Name: Amaranth
Botanical Name: *Amaranthus hypochondriacus*

The active properties of this plant are classed as astringent and nutrient. The plant contains generous amounts of vitamins and minerals, and it has been used in different parts of the world as a pot herb.

For centuries, the Chinese and various other peoples have employed amaranth as a remedy for profuse menstruation. Two ounces of the herb are placed in a container, and one quart of boiling water is poured on. The brew is covered, allowed to stand until cold, and then strained. The tea is reheated to take the chill off, and one large cup of the lukewarm tea is taken four or five times a day. (In more severe cases, the tea may be taken more often.)

Reported Uses

• A young married woman wrote:

"The flow of my periods was so heavy that I couldn't go out of the house during the first three days of my monthly period. Different medications gave no relief, then someone suggested an herb tea called Amaranth. I was unfamiliar with Chinese herb remedies, but was willing to try anything that might help. I began drinking several cups of the tea daily for the first few days of my period. It was amazing that something so simple could help so much . . . the flow was reduced to normal. Now I take the tea regularly on those days of the month and have never had any further trouble."

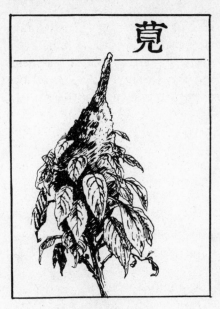

HSIEN
(Amaranth)

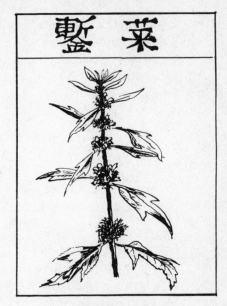

TSAN-TS′AI
(Motherwort)

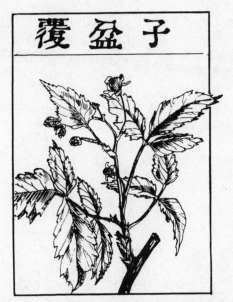

FU-P′EN-TZU
(Red Raspberry)

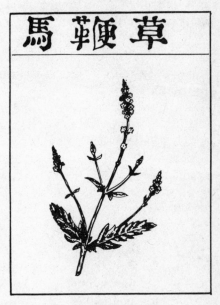

MA-PIEN-TS′AO
(Vervain)

• Miss R.V. gives this account:

"My problem was excessive menstruation. It got so bad that I had to be off work the first two days of every monthly period. Drinking amaranth herb tea regulated the flow so I no longer lose any time at work, nor do I dread the approach of menstruation anymore."

FU-P'EN-TZU

English Name: Red Raspberry
Botanical Name: *Rubus strigosus*

The common raspberry grows in many parts of the world, including the uplands of the central and western provinces of China. Its Chinese name, Fu-p'en-tzu, means "a turned-over bowl," in reference to the shape of the fruit. A number of other names are given, some of which apparently refer to the foreign origin of the plant.

In Chinese medicine a tea prepared from raspberry leaves is recommended as a female tonic and restorative. It is employed to help prevent miscarriage, to relieve the severe labor pains of childbirth, and to treat urethral irritation and menstrual difficulties. One cup of the tea, prepared as an ordinary tea, is taken three or four times a day for profuse or painful menstruation and for urethral irritation.

To ease the pains of childbirth and to help prevent miscarriage, one ounce of dried raspberry leaves is placed in a porcelain container, and one pint of boiling water is poured over. The tea is covered with a lid and allowed to stand until cold, then strained and reheated. One small cupful is taken half an hour before each meal.

Modern Support of the Ancient Chinese Claims

• Dr. Kirschner states:

"Herbalists have long prescribed raspberry leaf tea during pregnancy. Medical men laughed at this 'superstition.' Then came the confession by a woman physician, Violet Russel, M.D., who wrote in the London medical journal *Lancet:* 'Somewhat shamefacedly, I have encouraged expectant mothers to drink this infusion. In a good many cases labor has been easy and free of muscular spasms.' "

Dr. Kirschner gives these instructions: "During confinement, a pint of raspberry leaf tea is taken daily. Ordinary dosage is 10 to 20 ounces of the hot tea made from an ounce of the dried leaves steeped in 20 ounces of boiled water. Sweeten with honey."[1]

• *Potter's New Cyclopaedia of Botanical Drugs* cites the following: "Dr. Thompson and Dr. Coffin recommended the drinking of raspberry leaf tea by pregnant females for giving strength and rendering parturition easy and speedy. It should be taken freely before and during confinement."[2]

• In reference to the use of raspberry leaf tea, Dr. Fox wrote: "It is an excellent remedy in painful and profuse menstruation and to regulate the labor pains of women in childbirth. A teacupful of strong red raspberry leaf tea, in which the juice of an orange has been pressed, taken three times a day during the last months of pregnancy, will render labor easy when the hour of parturition has arrived."

• The following information appears in a Canadian book on herbs:

Red Raspberry Leaves: A good source of vitamins A, B, C, G, and E. They are rich in calcium, phosphorus, iron, and an unknown factor that prevents miscarriage. I know of several cases where this was proved beyond a doubt. A woman had four miscarriages, and despaired of ever bearing a child. Several doctors told her that she could never become a mother. On advice given by close members of my family, she took to drinking raspberry leaf tea every morning during pregnancy. She gave birth to a lovely girl, and in eighteen months she had another. The labor in both cases was practically painless.[3]

• J.H. Oliver, a medical herbalist of England, wrote: "A lady doctor who had been practicing for many years in a maternity home, and had helped thousands of babies into the world, told us she had always insisted on the prospective mothers taking raspberry leaf tea, and she scorned the idea of ever losing a case. Since we started this campaign we have received scores of letters from grateful parents. One lady told us she was reading the paper only a few minutes before her baby was born."

---

[1] *Nature's Healing Grasses*, p. 97.

[2] Wren, R.C., *Potter's New Cyclopaedia of Botanical Drugs* (London: Sir Isaac Putman & Sons, Ltd. 1956), p. 193.

[3] James, Claudia V., *Herbs and the Fountain of Youth* (Edmonton, Alberta, Canada: Amrita Books, 1959), p. 68.

• The following interesting account appeared in a health publication:

> A number of people find it difficult to relax when nervous or in pain, women particularly, especially during childbirth. The birth of my own first child was prolonged and frightening, mainly due to my fear and inability to relax the necessary muscles.
>
> Three years later, when I was pregnant again, I dreaded the coming ordeal. I had not, as yet, discovered the benefits of herbs. One day I was admiring a sow and litter with a neighboring farmer and remarked on the dreadfulness of producing such a large family. He laughed and told me that he always gave his sows an herbal remedy of raspberry leaf tea to help them when farrowing, and also thought that many ladies could benefit from the same herb.
>
> I was willing to try anything to allay my fears, and purchased a packet of raspberry leaf tea from a local herbalist. At first I did not care for its unusual flavor but in time I grew accustomed to it, and schooled myself to take it regularly. The months passed and the day came when I knew my baby would soon arrive. I was filled with an apprehension, which I soon found was quite unnecessary. My fears vanished when I found myself responding quite involuntarily to the muscular contractions with very little discomfort, and was amazed when the baby came into the world with such ease. My crowning achievement was a lovely little daughter whose quick arrival forestalled a surprised doctor who remembered my last drawn out ordeal.
>
> The practical experience with herbal treatment has strengthened my belief in the potential cures that are obtained from herbs. I have since learned that Dr. Grantley Dick Read advocated the use of raspberry leaf tea as an aid to easier childbirth in some of his studies of natural childbirth.
>
> So the farmer's recommendation proved successful; only someone who has suffered pain because of unrelaxed muscles can know the advantage of discovering a reliable source of help, and a simple one, too.
>
> I am fully convinced that I found such a remedy in raspberry leaf tea, and by taking it regularly throughout the latter months of pregnancy ensured myself of an easier birth.[4]

Fragarine

It is interesting to learn that during World War II the drug *fragarine* was discovered by obstetricians for use in allaying severe pains of childbirth. Fragarine is the active principle extracted from raspberry leaves and appears to relax the uterine muscles. It was

---

[4]*Fitness,* January 1963.

reported, however, that midwives ignored the new drug and continued to brew raspberry leaf tea for their patients.

Other Raspberry Leaf Formulas for Female Disorders

1. To relieve menopausal or menstrual "nerves," one ounce each of dried raspberry leaves and dried lime flowers *(Tilia europoea)* are mixed together. One teaspoonful of the combined herbs is placed in a cup, and boiling water is added. The cup is covered with a saucer, and the tea is allowed to steep for five minutes and then strained. One cup is taken three times daily.

2. For the condition of leucorrhea (a distressing complaint consisting of a whitish or creamy discharge from the mucus glands of the uterus) the following herbal formula is used. One ounce each of the *fluid extract or tincture* of raspberry leaves, gentian root *(Gentiana lutea)*, comfrey *(Symphytum officinalis)*, uva-ursi *(Arcto-staphylos uva-ursi)*, golden seal *(Hydrastis canadensis)*, are mixed together in one bottle. One teaspoonful of the combined fluid extracts or tinctures is taken in a little water three times daily after meals.

Accessory Treatment. In addition to taking the above formula, the cleansing process of an herbal douche is used. A mixture of one ounce each of raspberry leaves, white oak bark, *(Quercus alba)*, witch hazel leaves *(Hamamelis virginiana)*, black currant leaves *(Ribes nigrum)*, and cranesbill *(Geranium maculatum)* is boiled slowly in two quarts of water for twenty minutes and then strained through a cloth. The straining process should be continued until the liquid is perfectly clear, and when the solution is cooled to a tepid warm it is used as a douche.

When the tip of the douche bag is inserted, the lips of the female organ are held snugly together with the fingers around the base of the tip. The herbal solution is then allowed to flow in, and as it does so it opens and washes thoroughly all the deep folds and crevasses. When a slight stretching sensation is experienced, the lips of the female organ should be released, allowing the herbal douche to flow back out again freely. As this occurs, the vagina returns to its natural folds again. This process is repeated several times, until the herbal solution has been used up. A fresh batch should be prepared and used every other night until the condition has cleared up. Some cases respond favorably after only one or two douches; others require longer treatments of a week or ten days and even longer. However, once the leucorrhea has stopped the douches should not be continued.

TSAN-TS'AI

English Name: Motherwort
Botanical Name: *Leonurus cardiaca*

This plant is native to the Far East and Europe, but has been naturalized in other lands. For centuries it has been valued by the Chinese as a remedy for various ailments, especially for weakness and disorders of the female, hence its common name of "motherwort." It reputedly has a good effect on the womb and tones and strengthens the uterine membranes and other female organs. It is used as a remedy for inflammation or irritation of the uterus and also for suppressed or retarded menses.

Motherwort is prepared as a tea. One pint of boiling water is poured over one ounce of the herb. The container is covered, and the tea is allowed to stand for one-half hour, then strained. One hot cupful is taken four times a day.

Combined Formulas

1. For nervous disorders that are peculiarly female, such as menopausal "nerves" and irritability, one-half ounce each of motherwort, passiflora *(Passiflora incarnata)*, lady's slipper herb *(Cypripedium pubescens)*, and valerian *(Valeriana officinalis)* are mixed together and placed in a porcelain container. One quart of boiling water is poured over the mixture, the container is covered, and the brew is allowed to stand for twenty minutes and then strained. One cupful of the tea is taken four times daily.

2. For suppressed menstruation, one-half ounce each of motherwort, boneset herb, dried parsley, and feverfew *(Chrysanthemum parthenium)* are mixed together and simmered slowly in one quart of water for twenty minutes. The tea is then strained and taken hot, one cup four times daily.

T'AO

English Name: Peach
Botanical Name: *Prunus persica*

The peach is native to China, a fact which is shown by the Chinese character representing it, which is one of the few unchanged ancient characters. The wood of the tree was used in ancient times for fortune telling. This is indicated by the way the Chinese character is composed—the right hand part meaning "omen," and the left part meaning "wood."

In ancient folklore the flowers of the peach tree were believed to possess supernatural powers that could drive away demons of ill health. Slips of peach wood were used as charms against evil spirits. The slips were worn on the person, attached to the door of the home, or set around the rooms of the house.

Used in Chinese Medicine

Many different parts of the peach tree—such as the bark, leaves, flowers, and so on—are prized in Chinese medicine for treating various ailments. For example, a strong tea made from peach leaves is said to be a very good remedy for relieving or preventing morning sickness (vomiting during pregnancy). Two to four tablespoons of the tea are taken first thing in the morning, and the same dosage is continued, if necessary, every one or two hours, or oftener. It is said that in most cases the remedy acts very promptly to bring relief.

The tea may be prepared the night before. One pint of boiling water is poured over one and a half ounces of dried peach leaves. The container is covered with a lid, and the tea is allowed to stand until cold. It is then strained and stored overnight in the refrigerator. In the morning the tea is reheated and taken warm according to the dosages previously cited.

Other Remedies for Morning Sickness. Here are a few of the many other Chinese remedies that have proved helpful in allaying the morning sickness of pregnancy:

1. A cup of ginseng tea, made from an instant ginseng tea bag, is sipped slowly first thing in the morning. This may be repeated in an hour or so if necessary.
2. Some women have found relief by drinking a tea made by steeping two tablespoons of oats in a pint of boiling water. The container is covered, immediately removed from the burner, and allowed to stand for thirty minutes. It is then reheated, and one teacupful is sipped every one or two hours until results are obtained. This is regarded as a very fine formula.
3. In some cases, sipping a glass of lemon juice in water first thing in the morning has proved helpful.

4. One or two cups of tea made from the leaves or blossoms of the herb yarrow *(Achillea millefolium)* has been known to check the nausea of morning sickness within minutes. The tea is prepared in the usual way—one ounce is placed in a container and one pint of boiling water added. The infusion is covered, immediately removed from the stove, allowed to stand for fifteen minutes, and then strained.

CHIANG

English Name: Ginger
Botanical Name: *Zingiber officinalis*

Ginger is reputed to be of value in relieving suppressed or retarded menstruation. One-half ounce of the powdered root is stirred in one pint of boiling water. One cup of the hot tea is taken three or four times a day (the tea is sipped slowly).

Combined Formula

Ginger combined with other herbs is used for the relief of ovaritis, a condition fairly common among women. Symptoms generally include tenderness or pain on the lower side of the abdomen just above the groin. One or both sides may be affected.

Usually the pain begins two or three days before menstruation and persists through the menstrual period, then gradually ceases or suddenly stops when the period has ended. If the condition continues every month, it is chronic and can affect the general health.

As a remedy for ovaritis, one-half ounce of ginger root and one ounce each of motherwort, feverfew *(Chrysanthemum parthenium)*, and pleurisy root *(Asclepias tuberosa)* are mixed together and boiled slowly in one quart of water for fifteen minutes. (Keep the container covered.) The decoction is then strained, and a half teacupful is taken warm every two hours during the day. As the condition improves, the dose is reduced to three times a day. The treatment should be continued (generally three or four months) until the periods are normal.

JENSHEN

English Name: Ginseng
Botanical Name: *Panax schinseng*

For leucorrhea, one ounce each of ginseng, black cohosh *(Cimicifuga racemosa)*, gentian *(Gentiana lutea)*, and golden seal *(Hydrastis canadensis)*, all in coarse powder, are mixed together and placed in one quart of brandy. The bottle is capped and shaken thoroughly for about one minute, then stored in a cool dry place for ten days. During this ten day period the bottle is shaken every day for one or two minutes. After the ten days have elapsed, the herbal tincture is strained through a muslin cloth. If any sediment remains, the straining should be repeated until the liquid is clear. Filter papers may be used instead of the muslin, but the straining process will take much longer.

Dose: Two tablespoonfuls of the herbal tincture are taken in a little water three or four times a day.

Accessory Treatment. The same herbal douche is prepared and used according to the directions given in the information covering the herb raspberry.

SUAN

English Name: Garlic
Botanical Name: *Allium sativum*

The Chinese have used garlic to treat many different conditions of ill health. They claim the bulb contains valuable healing properties, even antiseptic powers. It is not surprising therefore to find that the Chinese sometimes recommend the bulb for certain female disorders such as menstrual cramps and vaginal infection. That some women have found this natural remedy effective can be seen by the following examples:

• Mrs. M.E. writes:

"I've always had menstrual cramps the first two days of my period. But ever since taking garlic (for about three months) I have very minor cramps. It's hard to believe, but it is the only thing I'm taking that I didn't take before that time. Now on each day of menstruation I take four or five garlic pills. I take two or three every day and, as said before, four or five on those difficult days."

• Another woman gives the following interesting account: "I am only twenty-three years old, but for five years I suffered from an agonizing vaginal yeast infection. I saw a total of four doctors, the last one being a specialist. They gave me every remedy from purple dye to strong antibiotics, and at the same time, believe it or not, the good doctors told me antibiotics can cause yeast infection by killing off the good bacteria as well as the bad. (As a child I had much sulfa and penicillin medication for ear infection).

"After reading that garlic acts like an antibiotic, I began to take fresh garlic cut up and, later on, manufactured garlic pills. I have found that, as with an antibiotic, when I discontinue the garlic, the infection starts again. But there are two distinct advantages of taking the garlic (combined with vinegar douches) over the doctor-prescribed antibiotics. It is much cheaper and there are no side-effects on the health of the rest of my body."

Note: A vinegar douche is prepared with four tablespoons of white vinegar to two quarts of warm water.

MA-PIEN-TS'AO

English Name: Vervain
Botanical Name: *Verbena officinalis*

The "Holy Vervain" or verbena is not to be confused with the lemon-scented verbena of gardens. It is, rather, a common plant with no aroma which bears small purple flowers.

Vervain reputedly contains natural properties which strengthen the womb and its appendages. It is said to cleanse and tone the lining of the womb and uterus and to free certain obstructions that interfere with efficient liver functioning.

Chinese herbalists have been aware of how dilation of arteries of the brain, which results in torturous migraine headaches or chronic headaches, can sometimes be traced to uterine and ovarian derangement. Although any one of a number of other causes could be the culprit of migraine, in those cases in which certain female disorders are responsible the herb vervain has often proved helpful.

To prepare the tea, instant vervain tea bags may be used or a quart of boiling water may be poured into a porcelain bowl containing two ounces of vervain. The bowl is covered with a lid, and the tea is allowed to steep for ten minutes and then strained. The whole quart is taken in teacupful doses throughout the day.

Reported Uses

• Mrs. M.B., who suffered vicious attacks of migraine headaches, writes: "I had to lie in bed in complete darkness for two whole days, and whatever tablets I took made no difference whatever.

"But life had to go on, and if I got up before my time the sickness was intensified. My husband would have to stay at home away from work, but there was nothing he could do except be at hand, downstairs. He had to prepare his own meals. To me, food was impossible.

"I used to enjoy having friends at the house and joining social activities, but I dared not face it any longer. Some friends thought I was making a lot of fuss about nothing.

"It was only after six years of torture that I discovered the effective relief in a simple infusion of vervain *(Verbena officinalis),* an herb popular as a health tizane on the continent and elsewhere, which can be obtained in small sachets sufficient to make a teacupful. I took several teacupsful daily."

SUMMARY

1. There are a number of different ailments that may affect the human female.
2. Menopause can leave a woman prone to a variety of unpleasant symptoms such as hot flashes, menopausal blues, and menopausal arthritis.
3. The change-of-life also means change of sex glands and thyroid gland.
4. Chinese girls are taught early in life the value of specific herbs to improve female health the natural way. They are also taught a few words of warning about the adverse effects of anything cold on the female system.
5. Dong Quai root has been famed for ages in Chinese medicine for its affinity for the female constitution.
6. Only the upper parts of Dong Quai, from the hip to the head of the root, are used as a domestic remedy.
7. Chinese Dong Quai is available in a powdered form prepared from the upper parts of a single root and as a stronger compound powdered form prepared from the upper parts of several roots. Preparations from the single root are milder and can be taken more often during the day. The stronger compound can be taken daily in lesser amounts.
8. For best results, little or no fruit should be eaten while you take Dong Quai, nor should any other type of strong root teas, such as ginseng, be taken for two or three hours after. Vegetables should

be included in the diet and should always be cooked with a slice of ginger root to maintain proper Yin-Yang balance.

9. When you drink herb teas for treating leucorrhea, herbal douches are always included as an accessory treatment.

10. There is a good variety of harmless Chinese herbs or herb formulas from which to choose for treating or relieving a wide range of female disorders.

11

CHINESE HERB REMEDIES FOR BOWEL COMPLAINTS

Mrs. L.L. suffered from internal "piles," symptomized by rectal itching and burning, a dull aching sensation, and pain up inside the rectum, with occasional bleeding. The pain increased during a bowel movement and became intensified when there was constipation. She reported:

"Surgery was advised, but I dreaded the knife, so I began checking into different forms of natural healing methods. My search led me to a Chinese herbalist, who gave me a box of capsules containing the powdered root of an herb he called *Collinsonia*, which I understand is also commonly called 'stone root' herb.

"He explained that Collinsonia was one of the most highly valued Chinese herb remedies for piles. He went on to say that generally two capsules taken twice daily between meals until results are obtained are sufficient for most cases. But since my condition was a bit worse than average he advised that I take two capsules three times a day between meals, and that as soon as definite improvement was noted, I should cut the dosage down to two capsules twice daily until cured. To immediately ease the rectal pain, burning, itching, and occasional bleeding until the healing treatment of Collinsonia could clear up the condition, he gave me a box of soothing herbal suppositories prepared from witch hazel and pilewort herb *(Ranunculus ficaria)*. A suppository was to be inserted night and morning and after each bowel movement.

"The herbalist also instructed that I keep my bowels open and suggested several helpful natural aids such as a baked apple or stewed prunes for breakfast. He cautioned me to avoid any fruit that had small seeds, such as figs, and also to avoid nuts since these things are not easy to digest and will often aggravate the condition of piles. However he added that nuts would be all right to eat provided they were finely ground and mixed with honey for use as a spread.

"Hygiene was also stressed. Coarse or scented toilet paper was not to be used. I was also instructed to bathe the anus with warm water after each bowel movement, dabbing dry with a soft towel set aside for this purpose.

"I followed all his instructions faithfully, and the results were just wonderful. Within several weeks, my condition was completely cured and has remained so from that time on (about two years). One unexpected and astonishing result was that the capsules of powdered Collinsonia root, in addition to curing my pile condition, also brought about marked improvement in the varicose veins in my legs!"

What Are Piles?

The word "piles" is the common name for the medical term *hemorrhoids*. It is a very annoying ailment which has plagued many people of all ages and either sex, although it is rare in the very young. The pain may range from simple discomfort to excruciating agony.

Medics inform us that piles are caused when the upward flow of blood through the rectal membrane is obstructed. Impeding the flow of blood up through the portal vein allows the remaining blood to congest in the veins of the rectum. If the condition continues, the walls of the veins lose their tone and become distended. This distension of blood vessels can be external, often causing the piles to protrude below the rectum. The condition of external piles can be seen and felt on the outer rim of the anus. The hemorrhoid can range in size from that of a small pea to that of a walnut. As much discomfort can often be experienced from a small external pile as from a large one.

The distension of blood vessels can be *internal* when the mucous membrane inside the rectum is the only part affected. With the condition of internal piles there is invariably a group of veins and arteries involved. The blood vessels are in a varicosed condition and are able to expand or contract according to the amount of blood which is congested in the rectum at any particular time.

If the internal pressure becomes great, the small veins of the rectal membrane can burst, causing a discharge of blood. This discharge relieves the congestion and brings prompt relief to the sufferer, but unfortunately such bleeding can sometimes be so frequent and profuse that the victim develops anemia. (Bowel movements may irritate the swollen veins of internal or external piles and also cause them to bleed at times.)

Many Causes

There are a number of different causes of obstruction of the upward flow of blood, which results in piles. One obvious cause is constipation. But this does not mean that costiveness must automatically lead to piles. If blood circulation in the rectum is strong and the walls of the rectal veins are firm and elastic, constipation will not lead to piles, unless there is also a circulatory obstruction in the vein abdominal flow. But if there is weakness in the rectum, the pressure of excrement contained there and in the lower part of the descending colon would tend to flatten the blood vessels by distending the membranes.

Examples of other causes are straining due to constipation or constant looseness of the the bowels, improper diet, other rectal troubles, or constant straining to urinate as in conditions of cystitis. Another important and common cause of hemorrhoids is congestion of the liver. Pressure upon the big portal vein leading to the liver would cause any blood that could not force its way past the constricted part of the vein to be held back in the rectal veins, allowing them to fill up with congested blood to produce piles.

The Action of Collinsonia Root

In view of all the facts outlined regarding the causes of piles, we can understand why the Chinese value the Collinsonia root as one of their most important remedies for hemorrhoids when we compare the facts to the following information from Ellingwood's *Materia Medica and Therapeutics:*

> Physiological Action: Collinsonia stimulates the stomach. It is actively tonic in its influence upon the entire function of this organ, and from this influence its beneficial action is exercised upon the *function of all vital organs. It is conspicuous in its ability to overcome relaxed and out of tone conditions of the walls of the veins. It has a direct influence upon atonic and dilated or otherwise impaired conditions of the veins and venous capillaries.* (Italics added.)

The action of Collinsonia root as pointed out by Ellingwood covers the basic cause of piles. The liver would benefit if the function of all the vital organs is improved, and most portal vein obstruction in the liver would be relieved. Regarding the action of the remedy upon the atonic and dilated veins, we find that Collinsonia identifies itself exactly with the condition the Chinese seek to cure.

Many Different Forms of Piles

In addition to Collinsonia root, the Chinese have a variety of other herb remedies for treating the early stages, and sometimes the advanced stages, of general hemorrhoid conditions, some of which are covered in the following pages. However, there are many types of piles of a very complicated nature which are beyond the scope of this chapter and which should receive the personal attention of a physician or practicing Chinese medical herbalist. Some examples are piles with prolapse of the rectum, ulcerated piles or piles with ulcerated rectum, internal piles complicated by colitis, piles with fissures, and so on.

Constipation

Simply defined, constipation means that bowel action is irregular, occurring only at prolonged intervals, or that bowel evacuations are excessively hardened and difficult to pass.

Along with food wastes, the bowels discharge cellular debris of body tissues, living and dead bacteria, mucus, and so on. When retained for longer than the normal period in the bowels, this mass of decaying debris offers a habitat and breeding ground for many harmful germs. These heated, putrefying wastes cause bowel discomfort, repulsive breath, sour stomach, headache, and other distresses associated with constipation. Poisons generated by putrefying wastes become a potential hazard to linings of the intestines. A feeling of depression and of "being out-of-sorts" have been blamed on irregularity.

Kellogg was of the opinion that the problem of constipation and associated autointoxication (a condition resulting from absorption into the blood stream of toxic fecal waste products due to chronic constipation) are the causes of most human ailments.

After much study, Professor Metchnikoff, a Russian biologist and Nobel prize winner in physiology, concluded that many diseases which affect mankind are caused by toxic types of bacteria which propagate in the large intestine. He further maintained that such intoxication is one of the chief causes of old age, and that its prevention would not only help man avoid many illnesses, but would also help preserve youth and prolong life beyond the so-called normal span.

"**Bathroom Straining**." Severe and repeated straining to move hard dry feces may cause fissures and/or piles. Straining at stool, of sufficient intensity and duration, also puts abnormal strain on the heart and threatens the life of any heart patient. According to a paper delivered to a symposium by Dr. Norman Shaftel, even people who have no signs of a heart problem can also dangerously over-burden their hearts when straining to move the bowels.

Dr. Shaftel reported that tests showed that straining produced important changes in blood pressure, heart rate, and electrocardio-graph patterns in people with no previous history of heart disorder. He said that such changes very closely resemble those which are observed in known heart patients.

Dr. Shaftel strongly recommended that physicians take every precaution to make sure their heart patients do not become con-stipated. Although he was unable to state just how frequently death has resulted from strained defecation, he did say, "It is not rare."

Writing in the *Journal of the American Medical Association* (September, 1961) Paul M. Zoll, M.D. points out that due to the increase in pressure within the thoracic and abdominal cavity while straining, "a diverticulum of the bowel, or an aneurysm of a major blood vessel of the left ventricle might rupture." He also warns that straining can bring on angina or "prolonged cardiac pain in a patient with extensive coronary disease."

Regularity—An Important Health Measure. Regular, normal bowel movements are important to help keep you feeling youthful and healthy. However, according to some authorities the "laxative habit" does more harm than good because the use of laxatives or cathartics (when taken in large enough doses to relieve stubborn constipation) irritates delicate intestinal membranes and interferes with digestion and absorption. In addition, laxatives may also cause cramps, diarrhea, and fluid depletion. Chinese herbalists agree with these views, and, although they readily admit that even concentra-tions of certain botanicals such as *senna* and other strong, stimulant type herbal laxatives are undesirable, they are quick to point out that the plant kingdom provides certain specific herbs and a large variety of natural foods that are not actually laxatives, but are *normalizers* and *regulators* of bowel function. They explain, for instance, that it is easier for the bowels to move if you include with your meals foods that contain roughage or bulk. Some examples are brown rice, oatmeal, buckwheat, unprocessed bran, and fruits and vegetables such as spinach, prunes, avocados, pumpkins, papayas, very ripe bananas, baked apples, and so on. By consuming ample portions of such foods and/or using one of a number of select Chinese herb teas, constipation can be overcome the natural way.

Exercise is also stressed. It is well known that people who spend any time in a hospital bed are frequently constipated, due to lack of exercise. Another of many examples is that of people who take long-distance vacation trips, driving steadily in their cars for hours at a time, day after day. Such people often complain of experiencing irregularity during their travels.

Daily exercise—such as a brisk walk, working in your garden, or riding a bicycle—is important to the maintenance of normal bowel activity.

Ample fluid intake is also important—at least six glasses of water should be taken a day, in addition to the liquids you normally consume with your meals. This would amount to well over one quart daily. The Chinese point out that when you do not drink enough fluid, the stool becomes dry, hard, and difficult to pass.

Diarrhea

Diarrhea is a condition of increased frequency and loose watery consistency of the stools. This can be a very serious and dangerous illness since it affects the mechanisms of the whole body. With diarrhea, the food does not remain long enough in the digestive tract to be absorbed. As a result, fats and carbohydrates are lost, and all the functions of these food elements in the body are not performed. All the work of calcium—which includes strengthening the bone and tooth structure, the heart, blood, and nerves—cannot be done since the calcium combines with the undigested fat and is carried away in diarrhea.

Prolonged diarrhea in infants and very young children can cause enough calcium loss to result in rickets; in adults it can cause bone softening. Loss of weight, poor appetite, and irritability are often due to the loss of calcium. Phosphorus, iron, potassium, many other valuable minerals, and the important fat-soluble vitamins A, D, K, and E are also sacrificed. And whenever there is a constant iron loss, anemia follows. A high incidence of respiratory ailments often occurs in patients suffering from diarrhea because their systems are depleted of vitamin A. (This vitamin is important in preventing infections and keeping the tissues healthy.)

In diarrhea cases blood sugar is also low, and the patient is left open to other physical disorders since blood sugar must be maintained at a certain level or exhaustion, weakness, allergies, blackouts, and other problems are likely to occur.

Dr. Carl L. Thenebe, a pediatrician, warns that when severe diarrhea strikes, body fluids, particularly the blood, become depleted of water. Demands are then made upon the cells of the body to make up the deficiency. When these cells become dry, a state of dehydration exists. When the body's water is lost there is, as previously stated, an outpouring of minerals or the electrolytes which are so essential to the life of the cell—calcium, phosphorus, iron, potassium, and so forth.

There are many causes of diarrhea. Dysentery, for example, is an inflammation of the large bowel and is symptomized by cramps, pain, and diarrhea. And there are many types of dysentery, each caused by a specific germ.

CHINESE HERB REMEDIES FOR BOWEL TROUBLES

Following is a list of natural Chinese remedies for coping with constipation, diarrhea, piles, and various other disorders of the bowels.

CHIN-CH'IAO-MAI

English Name: Yellow Dock
Botanical Name: *Rumex crispus*

Dock is the name applied to a wide variety of wayside plants such as Round-Leaved Dock, Water-Dock, and so on. They are found growing in ditches, meadows, and fields and are very common in China and other parts of the world. All docks are considered medicinally useful, but the species known as yellow dock *(Rumex crispus)* is the variety Chinese herbalists value most. This plant is easily recognized by its long narrow leaves which have crisp curled edges.

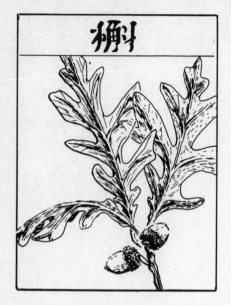

HU
(White Oak)

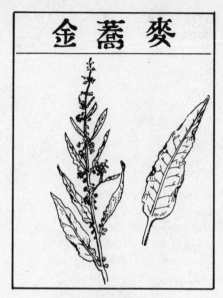

CH'IN-CH'IAO-MAI
(Yellow Dock)

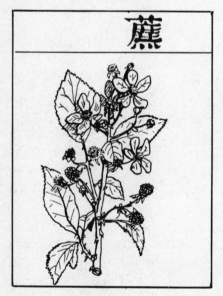

PIAO
(Blackberry)

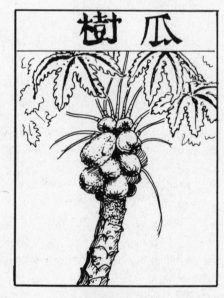

SHU-KUA
(Papaya)

Nature's Aid for Irregularity

A tea made from yellow dock is said to be a gentle natural aid for anyone troubled with constipation. The tea is not considered a laxative, but rather a normalizer and regulator of bowel function.

The root is the part of the herb used for making the tea. Although hard substances such as roots and barks are generally boiled continuously for a certain length of time in order to extract their active properties, delicate yellow dock root is an exception to this rule and must never be allowed to boil *continuously.* It is simply prepared by placing one teaspoonful of the cut roots in a cup and pouring on boiling water. The cup is covered with a saucer and allowed to stand for one-half hour. It is then strained, reheated, and taken hot. One cup of the tea is taken three or four times a day.

For the sake of convenience, a pint or quart of the tea may be prepared and one cupful at a time reheated for use during the day. One ounce of the cut roots is used to make one pint of the infusion; two ounces of the cut roots are used for one quart of the infusion. The cut roots are placed in a container. Using a separate container, bring one pint or one quart (as the case may be) of water to a boil and then pour it into the container which holds the cut roots. The tea is covered with a lid, allowed to stand for one-half hour, and then strained.

Individual Needs

The Chinese point out that the problem of constipation varies with different people, so that the amount of yellow dock tea taken daily depends upon individual needs. For example, some people may find that less than the average three or four cups daily is sufficient, whereas others may need more. The tea is perfectly harmless; it is a natural beverage. (Many people enjoy the bitter taste of yellow dock root tea, but for those who do not, the tea may be sweetened with honey.)

The Chinese also explain that with some people it may take a few days of drinking the tea daily before normal bowel function begins to take hold. Once it starts, irregularity is usually abolished from then on, so long as the tea is consumed daily thereafter. However, it is suggested that a daily enema should be used until the tea begins producing results. If the bowels still do not move after several days' use of the tea, some other natural remedy may be tried.

In very stubborn cases of constipation, the Chinese recommend that in addition to yellow dock root tea breakfast should consist of a natural food that helps normalize bowel action, such as a baked apple or a dish of stewed prunes topped with slices of a very ripe banana. Again, individual needs are stressed. When you use a natural breakfast food, only one or two cups of the yellow dock tea may be necessary—or more of the tea may be required. The only way to find out which is best for your own particular needs is to adjust the program accordingly.

Reported Uses

• "I suffered from constipation, and at times my bowels would not move for three or four days. Finally I had to take laxatives. I tried all kinds, but it was always the same old story of gripping pains, harshness, and the 'runs.'

"I was willing to try almost anything to get away from using laxatives, so when an acquaintance told me about a Chinese herb remedy called yellow dock tea, I decided to try it. The result was pure magic. I drink one cup of the hot tea first thing in the morning before breakfast and take three more cups during the day. I have done so for the past two years. Right from the second day on, I had regular bowel movements, just as normal as nature intended. There was no gripping, looseness, or harshness. Anyone troubled with constipation should know about this Chinese herb tea. It really works beautifully."—C.R.

• "When it comes to regularity, my hat's off to yellow dock root tea. Four cups of the tea taken daily cured my long-standing constipation. I used to get relief only from laxatives or enemas, but that's all in the past now. So long as I drink the herb tea daily, I have good healthy bowel movements."—Mr. T.L.

• "I would like to relate my husband's experience with a Chinese herb tea named yellow dock tea. For over a year, my husband didn't have normal bowel movements and had to use either physics or enemas. Yellow dock tea was the answer to his problem. He took three cups of the tea the first day, and when there was no result by the next two days he increased it to five. That did the trick. He had a natural bowel movement and has continued to have them regularly (about eight months now). He drinks the tea faithfully. Another remarkable thing is that he says the tea does not cause watery stools . . . the bowel movements are very natural."—Mrs. R.W.

• "My father, who is 72 years old, was troubled with constipation. Although many different laxatives and pills prescribed by the doctor were tried, they didn't really do the job, so finally he had to rely mostly on enemas.

"Thanks to a friend, we heard about yellow dock root tea. My father drank three large cups of the hot tea daily, and on the third day he had a partial bowel movement. He increased the amount of tea, but for several days he still had only partial movements. Nevertheless, he was very encouraged by the results and began following the additional instructions for stubborn constipation cases. He ate a dish of stewed prunes with sliced ripe banana for breakfast and drank the tea during the day. He had a complete normal bowel movement the following day.

"We were all as surprised as he was when he told us about it. As time went on, he found that by eating the natural breakfast food he could cut the tea down to two cups a day and still maintain daily regularity. One time he omitted drinking the tea for a few days because he was curious to see if the breakfast food alone would give the same good results. But he found the best it could do was produce partial movements, so he went right back to including the tea again. The combination resulted in the same complete daily regularity as before and has done so now for three years."—Mrs. C.B.

• "I suffered from miserable constipation and had to strain so hard that I developed painful piles. I hated taking laxatives since they not only irritated the pile condition, but also gave me the "runs." So on those days when I felt I just had to take a physic, I wouldn't go out anywhere for fear I'd suddenly get an urgent call from nature and might not have enough time to make it to a women's restroom.

"One day, instead of taking laxatives I began drinking yellow dock tea. I started with four cups, then increased it to five. Three days later I had a normal bowel movement, not loose or runny, but soft and natural. And there was no sense of sudden urgency to dash to the bathroom, but just nature's gentle way of letting you know, so you'd have plenty of time to heed her call. I was absolutely delighted and found that so long as I drank the tea daily I'd get the same fine results. And since there was no need to strain and I quit using laxatives, my pile condition cleared up within two weeks! I have been drinking yellow dock tea every day for about a year and a half and have never been constipated in all that time.—Mrs. V.R.

• "For years I was troubled with constipation. Five months ago, I threw out all the laxatives and started drinking yellow dock tea daily, and the result has been regular bowel movements ever since."—Mr. S.C.

HU

English Name: Common White Oak
Botanical Name: *Quercus alba*

There are more than forty species of the genus *Quercus* distributed widely over China, however, the identification of Chinese names are somewhat confusing because many of the different characters may apply to the same species or be used in combination with each other or with other characters in different parts of the country.

The species we are considering here is known as the common white oak tree. The acorns cluster in ones and twos and are attached to the twigs by long stems, the leaves having barely any stalks at all.

The bark is the part of the oak used in Chinese medicine, and its action is cited as slightly tonic, strongly astringent, and antiseptic. It is considered a good remedy for diarrhea and dysentery. A decoction is made with one ounce of the bark and two pints of water, boiled down to one pint and strained. One cupful is taken every one or two hours until relief is felt.

Capsule Form. Some people have reported very good results in abolishing conditions of diarrhea or dysentery by using white oak bark in powdered form contained in gelatin capsules. Two capsules are swallowed with a glass of warm water three or four times a day.

Other Uses of White Oak Bark

For mild conditions of colitis, one-half ounce each of oak bark, marshmallow root *(Althea officinalis)*, comfrey root *(Symphytum officinalis)*, slippery elm bark *(Ulmus fulva)*, sweet flag root *(Acorus calamus)*, and bayberry bark *(Myrica cerifera)* are boiled in three pints of water for ten minutes. The decoction is then strained. When it has cooled, it is bottled for use and stored in the refrigerator. Three to four teaspoonfuls are taken daily in a little warm water after meals, until results are obtained.

As an external treatment for bleeding piles, oak bark sitz baths are reputedly very effective. Six ounces of the bark are boiled slowly in one gallon of water for thirty minutes, then strained and decanted into a hip bath which is filled with cold water up to the usual level. This cold oak bark sitz bath is said to be wonderfully invigorating and has been described as a blessed relief from bleeding piles.

If the Spartan treatment of the oak bark sitz bath is undesirable, an injection of the cold oak bark decoction with a rectal syringe may be used instead. For this purpose, the decoction is prepared by simply adding one ounce of oak bark to one quart of water, and slowly boiling the mixture down to one pint. When cold, the decoction is strained through a muslin cloth and the liquid is used as a rectal injection. With the rectal syringe, inject about two ounces of the cold decoction into the rectum and retain for one hour if possible. If the bowels move, inject another two ounces and retain for an hour. The Chinese maintain that this treatment will strengthen the bowel and help relieve constipation, as well as arrest the bleeding of piles. It can be done every day until satisfactory results are obtained.

In addition to the external treatments for bleeding piles, a tea made from the herb pilewort *(Ranunculus ficaria)* is taken cold, in teacupful doses, four or five times a day. This herb has strong antiseptic qualities and is considered almost a specific for any type of piles, hence its popular common name of "pilewort."

The tea is prepared by placing one ounce of the herb in a porcelain container and pouring on one pint of boiling water. The container is covered and the tea allowed to stand until cold, then strained. It reputedly heals the majority of cases of piles in a few days.

TS'U

English Name: Vinegar

Other Chinese names for vinegar include Tso, Hsi, and K'u-chin. In China, different types of vinegar are made from various natural substances, such as rice, wheat, apples, cherries, peaches, grapes, and certain other fruits.

Among its uses in Chinese medicine, apple cider vinegar is recommended as a wash for pruritus of the anus. This is a chronic condition of itching of the anus (the final one or one-and-a-half inches of the rectum). The cause is usually of unknown origin, however, recent evidence has indicated that one of the possible causes is that some people are allergic to fresh or canned citrus juices, and if they are taken in other than very minute quantities, itching of the rectum (pruritus ani) results.

For best resuts, the vinegar is generally used full strength. However, it may be diluted with a little water. First the anal area is washed with clear water (no soap), then the area is thoroughly dabbed or bathed with a wad of cotton saturated with vinegar. (If the anus has been irritated by scratching, the vinegar will cause a temporary burning or smarting sensation.) The treatment is used once or twice a day until the condition is totally cleared up. Results are claimed to be very fast.

Reported Use

• Mrs. V.R. writes:

"For several months I suffered the unbearable itching of pruritus of the anus, with only mild and temporary relief from medical prescriptions. Then, by good fortune, I heard about a Chinese remedy of bathing the rectal area with vinegar. I soaked a large piece of cotton with ordinary vinegar and applied it to the rectum overnight. It brought complete relief, and there has been no further recurrence of the problem in over eight months. When I first applied the vinegar it smarted quite a bit, but the smarting lasted only for a few moments. It is still hard to believe how quickly this simple remedy worked and how very effective it was."

PIAO

English Name: Blackberry
Botanical Name: *Rubus fructicosus*

The root, leaves, and bark are all classed as astringents, but the root is more strongly astringent than the leaves or bark.

A tea made from blackberry root has long been used in Chinese herb medicine as a remedy for dysentery and diarrhea. The Chinese also maintain that it strengthens the Yin. This is interesting when we consider that diarrhea or dysentery has a weakening (Yin) effect on the body. Therefore, if the remedy corrects these conditions, the patient regains his strength; i.e., the Yin would be strengthened.

Blackberry root must be boiled for a long time in order to extract its astringent properties. For conditions of diarrhea, a decoction is prepared by placing two and a half ounces of the cut roots in one and a half quarts of water. The container is covered, and the decoction is brought to a boil and boiled very slowly (simmered) down to one quart. When cool, one cupful of the strained decoction is taken every two or three hours or one tablespoonful is taken every fifteen or twenty minutes, until relief is felt.

For a stronger formula for diarrhea, the decoction is prepared with milk instead of water. (The same amount of cut roots is boiled slowly, in one and a half quarts of milk, down to one quart and strained.) The dosage is the same as it was in the previous recipe.

For dysentery, one ounce each of cut blackberry roots, wild cherry bark, and white oak bark is mixed with the others and boiled slowly, in three pints of water, down to two pints. When cool, one half to one teacupful of the strained decoction is taken several times a day until results are obtained.

MAI-FU

English Name: Wheaten Bran

In China wheaten meal is of a very good quality since only tiny amounts of bran and wheat germ (high fiber food sources) are removed from the flour, due to the rough mode of grinding the meal. By contrast, for many years the mills of flour industries of Western nations have been removing all the bran and wheat germ from the flour by means of modern refining methods. As a result, a large number of scientific studies indicate that the lack of fiber in our diet has caused a prevalence of certain diseases relatively uncommon in China and other lands where high fiber foods such as bran, wheat germ, brown rice, and so on are still eaten. Some examples of such diseases cited include constipation, gall bladder problems, cancer of the colon, hemorrhoids, diverticular disease, and appendicitis.

How the Chinese Use Bran

As a domestic remedy, the Chinese use unprocessed bran in different forms. For example, bran mixed with vinegar is applied externally as a poultice for inflammation, boils, and so forth; a pillow stuffed with bran is used in place of an ordinary pillow for inducing relaxation in cases of insomnia; or bran made into a tea is used for profuse sweating and certain urinary problems. However, a daily ration of unprocessed bran in the diet is especially valued as an effective natural means of preventing or relieving constipation. For this purpose, the Chinese instruct that sufficient fluids—such as milk, soup, juice, or broth—should always be taken with bran. The bran may be stirred in the fluids, or, if the bran is baked into muffins, eating of the muffins should be accompanied by drinking of fluids. The reason for this is that bran has the ability to absorb many times its weight in water or watery fluids, and it is the fluid that makes the type of large, soft stools that pass easily.

Generally, two teaspoonfuls of unprocessed bran are taken three times a day, but some people find that less is sufficient, while others may need more. The Chinese explain that each person must find the amount suitable to his own individual need, and this may be done by starting with one or two teaspoonfuls of bran per day and gradually increasing the amount each day until the desired results are achieved, then continuing daily with that specific amount. White flour and refined sugar should be greatly reduced in the diet.

Centuries of experience have convinced the Chinese that unprocessed bran is not a laxative, but rather a normalizer of bowel elimination, and therefore is of value not only in conditions of constipation, but also in troublesome diarrhea.

However, they point out that some people find that when they add bran to their diet it causes temporary discomfort from flatulence. But in most cases the problem disappears within two or three weeks. And a few people may find that bran disagrees with them. In such cases, other types of natural high fiber foods and/or specific herb teas such as yellow dock may be the answer to their constipation problem. The Chinese add a word of caution that any food source high in dietary fiber, such as bran, should not be used for constipation by patients with intestinal stenosis or adhesions.

Bran sold in supermarkets is generally processed and usually contains sugar. Unprocessed bran (the type of bran used by the Chinese) can be obtained from health food stores and various herb firms.

Some Scientific Findings on the Value of Bran

As early as 1941, Surgeon Captain Cleave of the British Royal Navy began reporting in medical literature on the value of unprocessed bran as one of the best and natural ways to cure or prevent constipation. In the *British Medical Journal* (May 1972), Cleave reviewed some of his past experiences and related that on one occasion while he was serving on a battleship there was a scarcity of fresh vegetables and fruits, and he found "bran invaluable for correcting constipation of the ship's company." He added, "The sailors loved the stuff by comparison with purgatives [very strong cathartics]. I think it is a great tragedy of our present age that, with Medical Research Council workers showing at least 15 per cent of the population to be on regular purgatives, this precious material [bran] is ever lost through the manufacture of white flour."

In a letter printed in a British medical publication, *The Lancet,* Dr. Harold Dodd wrote: "Constipation is an ailment of so-called civilization and it can be greatly relieved by the way we live. I cannot speak too highly of Surgeon Captain Cleave's prescription—one tablespoonful of unprocessed bran daily. It restores to the diet what the miller has taken out. For several years I have practiced and prescribed a dessertspoon of unprocessed bran and one of unprocessed wheat germ daily. It is moistened according to taste with milk, gravy, soup, coffee, or fruit juice. In most patients it ensures a daily formed stool as smooth as with liquid paraffin."

Dr. Neil S. Painter, a London surgeon, and his colleagues engaged in a long-term study in which they gave bran to patients with diverticulosis. They reported the results in an article entitled "Unprocessed Bran in Treatment of Diverticulosis Disease of the Colon," which appeared in the *British Medical Journal* (April 15, 1972). In this study, anywhere from one teaspoonful to nine tablespoonsful of unprocessed bran were taken daily by seventy patients with diverticular disease, each patient adjusting the dose to his own personal comfort. Most of the patients took their bran with milk, soup, or water or sprinkled on cereals, the average dose being two teaspoons three times a day. In addition to the bran, Dr. Painter also placed his patients on a high residue diet—including whole meal bread, vegetables, fruits, and porridge—and advised them to cut down on sugar.

Of the sixty-two patients who continued the program faithfully every day, 90 per cent were able to relieve or completely abolish their symptoms, which ranged from severe colic to nausea, heartburn, tender rectum, bloated feeling, and constipation. Whereas about 80 per cent of the patients previously had to strain and had stools that were small and hard, their bowels now were regular, their stools were large and soft, and they no longer needed to strain. Patients with the opposite problem also were helped. Prior to using bran, one individual needed to visit the bathroom six times a day, and another did so twelve times a day. However, on the bran diet each had only two bowel movements daily. (Other researchers have reported the same effect, which indicates that bran is a *normalizer* of bowel elimination.)

Dr. Painter reported that his findings also suggest that "the widely held view that so-called 'roughage' irritates the gut is not founded on fact; bran, when moist, becomes 'softage.'"

However, another medic, Dr. Marian T. Troy, adds a warning that if diverticulosis reaches the acute stage of diverticulitis, the dietary advice is different. Dr. Troy explains that this is a very painful inflammatory disease, not a condition, and when it is in the acute state the old fashioned advice of a low-residue or no-residue diet applies. She goes on to say, "If you should suffer a bout of diverticulitis, drink only clear liquids, but no milk. You want your bowels to be empty, to let the inflammation subside, to let any pus in the diverticula drain into the bowel. Do not try to treat a bout of diverticulitis yourself. This is a job for your doctor." She advises that to avoid diverticulosis in the first place, you should eat green vegetables, fresh fruits, and some unprocessed bran every day and cut out highly refined foods.

Other research studies on the value of unprocessed bran were reported in the *Medical World News* (Sept. 6, 1974). These studies pointed to the ability of bran to lower cholesterol and to help prevent cardiovascular disorders—such as occlusive vascular diseases, ischemic heart disease, deep vein thrombosis, and varicose veins—and other conditions related to metabolism, such as diabetes and obesity.

P'ENG

English Name: Canada Fleabane
Botanical Name: *Erigeron canadense*

The medicinal action of this plant is cited as tonic and astringent. It is used in cases of diarrhea and dysentery. It is prepared as a tea. Two pints of boiling water are poured over two ounces of cut pieces of the herb. The container is covered, and the brew is allowed to stand for one-half hour and then strained. The tea is taken cold, one cupful every hour or two until relief is achieved.

If a fluid extract of the herb is used in place of the tea, one-half to one teaspoonful of the extract is added to a small glass of cold water, and the mixture is taken until results are obtained.

The Chinese were not the only ones who valued Canada Fleabane for conditions of diarrhea. The North American Indians and early settlers also used the herb for the same condition. In the *Journal of Allergy* (September, 1955), J.A. Blue, M.D. reported that when Indians and early settlers suffered the sometimes serious problem of diarrhea, they relied on a tea made from Canada Fleabane. In reference to the herb, Dr. Blue said that experiments showed that it worked when diarrhea "proved so baffling and defied the best modern remedies to relieve it."

YU

English Name: Slippery Elm
Botanical Name: *Ulmus fulva*

There are many varieties of elm. Slippery elm is a small tree with rough branches and long leaves rough with hairs on both sides. A yellow "wool" covers the leaf buds. Flowers are stalkless.

The inner bark is the part of the tree used in Chinese medicine and is considered one of nature's most excellent demulcents and nutritives. It is employed for its ability to absorb foul gases in the body. It is also used for its gentle, soothing action in cases of enteritis (inflammation of the intestinal tract) and colitis (inflammation of the large bowel). There are many types of colitis. Some are mild, others are very severe.

Because of its soothing, mucilaginous nature, the use of slippery elm reputedly assures easy passage during the process of bowel evacuation. In addition it acts as a buffer against irritation and inflammation of the mucous membranes and is considered helpful in conditions of dysentery and diarrhea.

One cup of the tea is prepared from the powdered bark and a pinch of powdered golden seal and is taken three times a day. As an accessory treatment for bowel inflammation, dysentery, and other diseases of the bowels, a second batch of the tea is prepared in the same way and used as an injection with a rectal syringe (after the tea has been cooled to luke warm).

Further Instructions

The powdered bark of slippery elm is difficult to mix without forming lumps. To solve this problem, the tea is prepared by placing two teaspoonfuls of the powder in a jar and adding one-half cup of cold water. The jar is capped, and the mixture is shaken thoroughly. The mixture is then poured into a porcelain container, and one pint of boiling hot water and a pinch of powdered golden seal is added. The solution is thoroughly stirred until the powders are well mixed and dissolved.

The same procedure is followed when you prepare another batch for use as a rectal injection. If the solution is too thick to flow freely through the syringe, the tea may be diluted with a little more water.

CHINESE GINSENG HERB PRUNES

This is a preparation in which Chinese ginseng is blended with prunes. No preservatives or chemicals are added. It is used daily as a natural breakfast food. This product reputedly relieves constipation because it acts as a strengthener and normalizer of bowel function. Many people troubled with irregularity have reported very good results from the use of this natural food blend.

Chinese Ginseng herb prunes come packed in cellophane bags, and each bag is packed in a carton. They are sold by herb firms and health food stores.

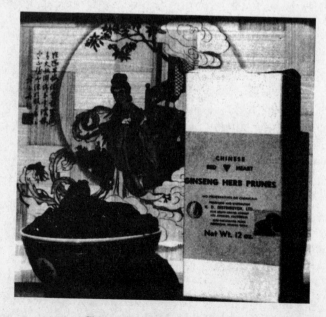

Chinese Ginseng Herb Prunes

SHU-KUA

English Name: Papaya
Botanical Name: *Carica papaya*

The papaya is a tropical melon-like fruit which is produced in clusters by the *Carica papaya* tree. In the tropics, where the papaya tree has been valued as a food and medicine for ages, fascinating stories and legends are told of the tree. In certain regions it is regarded by the natives as a mystical plant because in some ways it appears to possess human attributes—producing male and female flowers in separate plants, while the fruit, like the human embryo, develops in about nine months.

The papaya tree was introduced and cultivated in South China and other parts of the Far East less than a century ago. Its Chinese name, *Shu-kua,* means "tree melon." Other Chinese names include *Wan-shou-kau,* "longevity fruit"; *Fan-kua,* "foreign melon"; and *Mu-kua,* which is another way of saying "tree melon."

Constituents of Papaya

The papaya contains an abundance of vitamins and minerals. It also provides enzymes—the most important being papain, which greatly resembles pepsin in its digestive action. The natural papain enzyme is extracted from the papaya, made into tablets, and sold on the market—mainly as an aid for protein digestion.

Chinese Usage of Papaya

After the introduction of papaya into China, the Chinese quickly learned to appreciate the usefulness of the papaya in rendering meat tender, as well as its alimentary and medicinal qualities. With reference to irregularity, the Chinese maintain that ripe papaya fruit eaten daily is an effective natural means of abolishing constipation. Many people have attested to the truth of this Oriental claim, stating that papaya worked for them when all other natural means had failed.

Modern Chinese herbalists sometimes recommend papain tablets for treating external hemorrhoids, which in some instances has proved successful. Generally, one tablet is taken every three or four hours until the ailment has cleared up, which, when the remedy is effective, usually occurs within a week.

Reported Uses of Papain for External Hemorrhoids

• Mr. R.G. was one of several people who claimed to have avoided surgery for painful external piles, the condition having been successfully treated by using papain tablets as directed by a Chinese herbalist.

• It is interesting to find that a modern Occidental physician also found that papain tablets were effective in treating a case of external piles. Phillip J. Pollack, M.D. reported the case of a woman 52 years of age who suffered painful external hemorrhoids. Standard therapy—rectal suppositories, sitz baths, and bed rest—produced no response. Dr. Pollack then instructed the woman to take one papain tablet every four hours. In forty-eight hours "marked improvement" was noted in the patient. Swelling and pain both subsided. After three more days of the papain treatment, the improvement was considered complete. Surgery was not necessary.[1]

Note: Because the fruit is highly perishable, importation of papaya into the United States from tropical regions has been a problem. But recently arrangements were made to ship the melons from Hawaii to the mainland by jet planes. However, if you still find that fresh papayas are not always available at your supermarket, other forms—such as papaya juice, frozen papaya, and dried papaya— are readily available from health food stores and are considered good substitutes for fresh papaya. Papain tablets may also be obtained from health food stores or from herb firms.

SUAN

English Name: Garlic
Botanical Name: *Allium sativum*

Among its varied uses in Chinese medicine, garlic is employed for treating ailments such as diarrhea, dysentery, colitis, and other intestinal disturbances. Either the fresh garlic cloves or garlic in tablet form or capsules (perles) may be used.

In mild cases of diarrhea or dysentery, two garlic tablets are taken once or twice a day. In average cases, two tablets are taken three times a day. In persistent cases, two tablets are taken four or five times a day. A finely chopped clove of fresh garlic can be used,

---

[1]*Current Therapeutic Research,* May 1962.

taken three times a day between meals. The chopped garlic may be added to a cup of warm milk or a cup of soup, such as clear beef broth. If garlic capsules are preferred, generally, one to two capsules are taken three times a day. If needed, they can be taken four times a day.

If the method of the finely chopped fresh garlic is used, a mouthful of the garlic broth or soup is taken, and at the same time a little of the finely chopped garlic is scooped up from the cup and swallowed with the mouthful of milk or broth. This procedure is continued until the whole cup of garlic milk or broth has been consumed.

Garlic capsules or tablets leave no odor on the breath, but as everyone knows the strong odor of fresh garlic does linger on the breath. However, the odor of garlic cloves may be eliminated by eating a few sprigs of fresh parsley directly afterwards.

Reported Uses

• "I was terribly weakened and run-down from occasional bouts of diarrhea. Nothing my doctor prescribed helped very much. I finally followed the suggestion of my neighbor who told me she heard that the Chinese often make use of garlic to treat diarrhea, and that her friend was quickly relieved of the same condition I had by trying the garlic remedy. So I chopped up a clove of garlic very fine and stirred it in a cup of warm milk. I took sips of the milk and swallowed some of the tiny pieces of garlic at the same time until the cup was empty. I did this between each meal. The diarrhea ceased almost immediately. Hope this information helps others as it did me."—Mrs. L.W.

• "Just recently, when a co-worker told me how he had suffered from diarrhea ever since the surgeon had removed hemorrhoids from him, I let him read a letter from someone who was helped by taking three garlic perles a day. He began taking some that I gave him, and they helped not only the diarrhea but his high blood pressure as well. And his blood pressure had been dangerously elevated. When his doctor checked him a few days ago, it was perfectly normal. He didn't tell him about taking the garlic perles, and neither did he get the prescription filled that the doctor had given him for the diarrhea."—T.L.

• "Some years ago I came across an interesting article in the *AMA Journal* while waiting in a doctor's office. It was an account of two young doctors who accidently discovered that garlic apparently killed harmful bacteria in the intestines while promoting the growth of beneficial bacteria. This was something no regular antiseptic or antibiotic could do. So I tried it, and it worked just fine. We have not had a case of diarrhea or any other intestinal disturbances in our family since then."—Mrs. I.M.

• "For the past year I have had repeated attacks of stubborn diarrhea. Then I tried garlic. I took two tablets three times a day, and after two weeks the condition was gone. This simple remedy worked far better than the medicine my physician had me take."—Mr. L.R.

• "I overcame dysentery with garlic tablets. They are good for so many other things that I always keep a supply on hand in the house."—Miss J.C.

Modern Science Studies Garlic

Medical reports from different parts of the world are gradually confirming many of the Chinese claims for the ability of garlic to cope with a wide range of ailments. Following are a few of many examples cited by qualified authorities with regard to the effectiveness of garlic in treating bowel and intestinal complaints.

1. Fusganger and Becher of Germany found that garlic was effective against intestinal putrefaction.

2. Emil Weiss, M.D., an American physician, wrote an article in the *Medical Record* (June 4, 1941) in which he described a series of experiments conducted on twenty-two patients. Every one of these subjects had well known histories of intestinal disorders. Several weeks before the experiments began, daily specimens of urine and feces were collected. The entire digestive processes of these patients were observed and carefully noted. The group of subjects was then divided, and garlic was given to one part of the group while the other part took no medication. During the garlic treatment, mild diarrhea, headaches, and other symptoms of intestinal trouble vanished. There was a complete change in the intestinal flora (bacteria living in the digestive tract) of those who had taken garlic. Some of these bacteria are very helpful, aiding with the digestion of food, while others are harmful, and their presence results in a condition of putrefaction and ill health. It was noted that at the end of the garlic treatments the harmful bacteria were decreasing while the beneficial ones were increasing.

3. T.D. Yanovich wrote an article describing his experiments with garlic.[2] He introduced garlic juice directly into the colonies of bacteria and found that all movement of the bacteria ceased within three minutes. He also added garlic juice to a culture of bacteria and found that this caused the bacteria to disperse to the edge of the culture. Immobile bacteria began to appear after two minutes and all activity had ceased within the short space of ten minutes.

4. Kristine Nolfi, M.D., of Norway, wrote of her medical experiences involving the use of garlic. In addition to citing its effectiveness in coping with a number of other disorders, she said it "kills putrefaction bacteria in the large intestine and neutralizes poisons in the organism itself."[3]

5. Professor Roos of Germany wrote an article in a medical magazine entitled *Munchner Medizinische Wochenschrift* (September 25, 1925) in which he mentions the medicinal value of garlic. His article mostly covers his experiences involving the use of garlic in treating a variety of intestinal disorders, and some remarkable case histories are cited. Here are some examples:

• A laboratory assistant accidently infected herself with a bacteria which causes dysentery. She developed alarming symptoms: no appetite, vomiting, diarrhea followed by bloody stools. She was weak, exhausted, and pain-wracked. This woman was given two grams of a garlic preparation five times a day for six days. Almost at once the vomiting stopped and she found she could eat again. On the 19th day the illness began to subside, but for quite some time before this she was able to be out of bed and felt cheerful.

Dr. Roos commented that: "I could not maintain that the length of time of actual illness was considerably shortened, only that convalescence transpired in a surprisingly rapid manner. To everyone experienced with cases of dysentery, the contrast must be extremely surprising between the obviously very severe form of the disease and the extremely light discomfort following introduction of treatment, along with only a mildly exhausted condition."

• A man 33 years old suffered from chronic colitis which manifested itself in frequent diarrhea, pain, and other unpleasant sensations. In the beginning he took two grams of garlic twice daily

---

[2]*C.R. de l'Academie des Sciences de l'USSR,* Vol. 8, No. 7 (1945).

[3]*My Experiences with Living Food* (Humlebak, Denmark: Humelgaarden), p. 11.

for fourteen days, then he took two grams of garlic once daily. Within the first few days he felt better. Three weeks after treatment began he had two normal stools daily.

• Two patients, age 36 and 47, suffered from gas, bloating, diarrhea, heart palpitations, and headaches. All symptoms were removed after they took garlic for six weeks.

• An inspector suffered from diarrhea, poor appetite, and gas. He had taken many drugs, but got no relief. By the end of the fourth week on garlic he was satisfied he was cured.

• A 23-year-old student complained of excessive gas, restlessness, loss of weight, a general feeling of ill health, and diarrhea. After taking garlic he returned to normal, with only one brief relapse.

• A patient complained that he had suffered from gas, dyspepsia, and colitis for seventeen years. Occasionally the diarrhea alternated with spells of constipation. He was given two grams of the garlic preparation two to three times daily. In two and a half months the patient considered himself cured.

• A patient had a case of nervous diarrhea. He suffered from this complaint whenever he became excited. The diarrhea was improved from time to time by the use of garlic. Dr. Roos notes that the patient came for the remedy quite often.

SUMMARY

1. There are a variety of bowel complaints which have yielded to the use of herb remedies and certain health measures.
2. Piles are symptomized by rectal pain, burning, itching, and sometimes bleeding. They can be internal or external.
3. "Bathroom straining" (repeated straining to move hard, dry feces) may cause fissures and/or piles. It also puts an abnormal strain on the heart.
4. The plant kingdom provides certain herbs and natural foods which help prevent or overcome constipation. They are not regarded as laxatives, but rather as normalizers and regulators of bowel functions.
5. Although hard substances such as roots and barks are generally prepared as decoctions (boiled for a certain length of time), delicate yellow dock root is an exception to this rule and must never be allowed to boil continuously. To allow it to do so would destroy the root's active properties.

6. Diarrhea and dysentery have a weakening (Yin) effect on the body. If such conditions are prolonged and are not corrected, they can be very serious and dangerous.

7. Among its varied uses in Chinese medicine, common garlic is employed for treating diarrhea, dysentery, colitis, and other intestinal disturbances.

12

CHINESE HERBS FOR COPING WITH HEADACHES, NERVOUSNESS, STRESS, AND INSOMNIA

For years Western civilizations have been drifting away from natural living and natural laws. Statistics show that an incredible number of people are taking tranquilizers, sleeping pills, and similar drugs for nervousness, insomnia, and stress. More often than not, the distressed patient is handed a medical prescription for some type of barbiturate drug, and many of these medicines produce side effects and are habit forming. Aspirin, the popular over-the-counter drug for relieving headaches, also causes side effects in many people.

According to a report by the U.S. Public Health Service, more accidental deaths result from an excess of barbiturates than from any other type of acute drug poisoning. Sometimes the continued use of sleep-inducing drugs brings about a trance-like state rather than genuine sleep. In such instances, the insomniac cannot remember exactly how many pills he has already swallowed so he takes more. This puts him to sleep permanently. In other cases, people make the dangerous and often fatal blunder of taking sleeping pills just before or shortly after drinking liquor. In analyzing twenty-one deaths caused by alcohol and barbiturate poisoning, two British pathologists concluded that the combination acts incredibly fast to produce a fatal drop in blood pressure.

The Chinese Method of Treatment

Chinese herbalists treat persons troubled with stress, tension, nervousness, insomnia, and nagging headache pains with specific herb remedies which are harmless and non-habit forming. Certain select herbs reputedly relieve various types of headaches; others help promote natural sleep; while still others feed and repair the worn nervous system, thereby helping to restore normal activity of the vital forces. However, due to the diversity of causes, a specific herb tea or formula may help one person but not another. Under the circumstances, it is best to select one herbal remedy and give it a sufficient trial. If after you have done so it does not help, you can switch to another. In this way you may be able to find the one most helpful for your own particular need. (It should also be noted that the limited space of one chapter necessarily prevents the listing of each and every Chinese herb remedy for the disorders cited.)

Along with the usage of herbs, the Chinese explain that Nature also requires sensible attention to the diet. Junk foods should be replaced by wholesome, well-balanced meals. And since food must have time to digest, you should never retire immediately after eating a meal. This practice has been known to cause nightmares or the stress and discomfort of prolonged restless twisting and turning in bed. Sufficient sleep is necessary so that energy used during the day can be restored to exhausted bodies.

The Chinese also advise that insomniacs cut down on salt in the diet.

CHINESE HERB REMEDIES

CHI-HSUEH-TS'AO

English Name: Catnip
Botanical Name: *Nepeta cataria*

Catnip herb belongs to the mint family and has a pleasant aromatic odor. It is reputed to be a good natural remedy for nervous irritability, nervous insomnia, and nervous headache when combined with other herbs and prepared as a tea. Following are some examples.

1. One teaspoon each of catnip, celery seeds, oats, valerian *(Valeriana officinalis)*, and scullcap *(Scutellaria laterifolia)* are mixed

together and placed in a container, and one and a half pints of boiling water are poured over them. The container is covered, and the tea is allowed to stand for twenty minutes. One warm cupful of the strained infusion is taken three times a day between meals, and one cupful is taken in the evening before you retire. The beverage is sipped slowly.

2. Another formula for treating nervous insomnia and nervous headache consists of one ounce each of catnip, scullcap, and peppermint. The herbs are thoroughly mixed and stored in a capped jar. One or two heaping teaspoons of the mixture are placed in a cup and filled with boiling water. The cup is covered with a saucer, the tea is allowed to stand until it is luke warm and then strained, and a teaspoonful of honey is added. .

For insomnia, one cupful is taken at bedtime. For nervous headache, one hot teacupful is sipped slowly every hour or two until relief is felt.

3. As a nerve tonic or a remedy for insomnia, one-half ounce each of catnip, scullcap, valerian, and passiflora *(Passiflora incarnata)* is mixed with the others and placed in a container, and one quart of boiling water is poured on. The container is covered, and the infusion is allowed to stand for twenty minutes and then strained. One teacupful is taken four times a day one hour after meals and about one-half hour before bedtime.

4. This combination may be used for nervous irritability or headache: One ounce each of catnip, sage, peppermint, and marjoram *(Origanum majorana)*, well mixed, is stored in a capped jar. One heaping teaspoonful of the mixture is placed in a cup filled with boiling water, the cup is covered with a saucer, and the tea is allowed to stand for five minutes and then strained. One cupful is slowly sipped every one or two hours until relief is felt.

LU-TS'AO

English Name: Hops
Botanical Name: *Humulus lupulus*

This is the common wild hop which is native to China, Japan, and many other lands. In Chinese it is called *Lu-ts'ao* and *Lai-mei-ts'ao*. Another Chinese name for the hops is *Le-ts'ao* because the stem of the plant is prickly and chafes the skin when it comes into contact with it.

The word *hop* is taken from the Anglo-Saxon *hoppen* meaning "to climb" because the twining perennial plant attaches itself to neighboring objects and attains a great height. The botanical name *Humulus* is derived from *humus,* "moist earth," the type of soil in which the plant thrives best.

Constituents and Medicinal Action

The active principle in hops is a glandular powder called *lupulin.* The peculiar fragrant odor is due to a volatile oil. The medicinal action of hops is cited as nervine, stomachic, tonic, soporific (induces sleep), and anodyne (relieves pain). For these reasons, hops are employed for nervous irritability, nervous sick headache, insomnia, neuritis, indigestion, and poor appetite.

In Chinese medicine hops are used in many different forms, such as teas, hop pillows, poultices, and fomentations.

The Hop Pillow—Nature's Sleep Aid

Centuries ago, hop pickers claimed that the strong aroma of the plant imparted a soothing, calming influence on the nerves. Pillows stuffed with hops were soon used in place of ordinary pillows to assure a good night's sleep in conditions of insomnia. As the years passed, their popularity spread to many other nations throughout the world, and they were even used by royalty. For example, records show that the use of a hop pillow was prescribed for George III in 1787, with excellent effect. It is also recorded that it was employed with very good results during an illness suffered by the Prince of Wales in 1879.

The soporific value of the hop pillow was mentioned in the 17th edition of the *U.S. Dispensatory:* "A pillow of hops has proved useful in allaying restlessness and producing sleep in nervous disorders. They should be moistened with water containing a trace of glycerin, previously to being placed under the head of the patient in order to prevent rustling."

Another method of preparing a hop pillow is to fill a muslin bag loosely with hops, tie the opening securely, and attach the bag to your regular pillow with a basting thread. Of course, the muslin bag (or pillow case) will need to be washed, and the hops should be renewed every month.

Note: Some people sprinkle the hops with a little alcohol, claiming it helps to bring out the soporific properties of the hops more fully.

Hops in Tea Form

Hop tea is used to relieve nervous insomnia, nervous irritability, and nervous headache. It is prepared in a covered vessel—one ounce of hops to one pint of boiling water. The tea is simmered for two or three minutes, removed from the burner, allowed to stand for five minutes, and strained.

For nervous irritability or insomnia, one hot teacupful is sipped three times a day and once before bedtime. In conditions of nervous sick headache, one hot teacupful is sipped slowly every two hours until relief is felt. The tea is also reputed to be an excellent tonic for the stomach, relieving indigestion and promoting the appetite. (Hop tea has an extremely bitter taste and may be sweetened with honey).

Combination Tea Formula

Hops are often combined with other herbs for use in conditions of nervous insomnia. One-quarter ounce each of hops, passiflora, and valerian is mixed with the others, and one pint of boiling water is poured over them. The container is covered, and the tea is allowed to stand for three hours and then strained. One cupful, reheated and sweetened with a teaspoonful of honey, is taken one-half hour before bedtime.

Hop Poultices and Fomentations

Hop poultices or fomentations are applied externally to relieve the pains of neuritis, which is an inflammatory condition of the nerves or nerve sheath. Doctors explain that although it can affect any part of the body, neuritis is generally situated in the main nerves of the face, leg, or arm. It may be caused by any number of things such as a cold, rheumatism, inflammation of some part of the body that also affects the nerves, or debility due to illness. Sciatica, facial neuralgia, and neuritis in the arm are all types of this disorder. When the sciatic nerve and branches are affected, the pain extends from the buttocks downward along the thigh to the knee and foot. When the arm is affected, the pain is felt from the back of the neck and top of the shoulder down the arm to the wrist or fingers. Sometimes there is a tingling or numb sensation. Facial neuralgia is symptomized by severe pains, generally on one side of the face.

Treatment

If the pain is in the face, the hop poultice or fomentation is applied in front of the ear or to the lower part of the back of the head. For pain in the buttocks and leg, the poultice or fomentation is applied approximately three inches from the base of the spine. When the pain is felt in the shoulder, arm, or fingers, the poultice or fomentation is applied to the upper part of the spine in line with the collar bone. These external applications placed on the specific areas mentioned, soothe the inflamed nerve where it branches out from the spinal cord.

How to Prepare Hop Poultices

A hop poultice is prepared by placing a large handful (or more) of hops in a muslin bag, tying the ends of the bag together with a piece of string, and steeping the bag in a covered container of hot water for a few minutes. When ready for use, the hop bag is quickly wrung out and applied, as hot as can be borne without causing a burn, to the specific area. The poultice is then covered with a folded dry towel to retain the heat as long as possible. In the meantime, a second poultice should be steeping in the hot water. As soon as the first poultice begins to cool, it is immediately removed and placed back into the container, while the second hot poultice is quickly wrung out and applied according to previous directions. The poulticing is continued in this manner until relief is obtained.

How to Prepare Hop Fomentations

If one prefers, fomentations may be used instead of poultices. In this case, a batch of hop tea is prepared in a covered vessel, with four ounces of hops to two quarts of boiling water. This is simmered for five minutes and then strained. A folded towel is dipped into the tea, quickly wrung out, and applied, as hot as can be tolerated without causing a burn, to the specific area. The wet towel is immediately covered with a dry one to retain the heat as long as possible. In the meantime, a second towel should be soaking in the hot tea (the vessel kept covered). As soon as the first towel begins to noticeably lose its heat, it is immediately removed and dipped back into the container of hop tea, and the second towel is wrung out and applied to the specific area. Fomentations are continued until relief is obtained.

Note: In using fomentations or poultices, the water or tea in the container should be kept hot during the entire period.

Accessory Treatment

One-half ounce each of hops, burdock, scullcap, valerian, and vervain *(Verbena officinalis)* are mixed together and half of the total mixture is placed in two pints of cold water and brought to a boil. The container is covered, and the decoction is simmered for ten minutes and then strained. It is taken warm, one tablespoonful several times a day. It reputedly soothes the inflamed nerves and gradually builds up the entire nervous system.

MA-PIEN-TS'AO

English Name: Vervain
Botanical Name: *Verbena officinalis*

As mentioned previously in the chapter on women's health, this plant is not to be confused with the lemon-scented verbena of our gardens. Vervain grows wild in low grounds, has no odor, and bears small purple flowers. When cultivated, the flowers reach a larger size. In Chinese the plant is given two different names, *Ma-pien-ts'ao* and *Lung-ya-ts'ao*.

Nerve Tonic

Medicinally, the herb has an ancient reputation as a strengthener of the nerves and for this purpose is generally prepared as a combined formula. Here is one of many such combinations. One ounce each of vervain, scullcap, and valerian are mixed together and three pints of boiling water are poured over them. The container is covered, and the tea is allowed to stand for twenty minutes and then strained. One warm teacupful is taken three times daily.

Headache Remedy

Vervain also has a long-standing reputation as a remedy for relieving various types of headaches—such as mild, congestive, or nervous-sick headache or those caused by fatigue or tension. One or two heaping teaspoonfuls of the cut, dried herb are placed in a teacup filled with boiling water. The cup is covered with a saucer, and the infusion is allowed to stand until cool. It is then strained and reheated. One teacupful is taken three or four times daily (or more often in severe cases) until relief is obtained.

In a few instances, this simple vervain tea has also brought relief from the pains of migraine headache. For example, a young man who had endured considerable stress stated he had suffered periodic bouts of migraine for years and it could not be cured. One day his family received a copy of a health magazine in which vervain tea was mentioned for the relief of migraine. He said, "I insisted on trying it. After the first few cachets of dried vervain in my tea, the migraine pains left and have not been felt since."

Although the tea will not help in every case of migraine, the Chinese claim it is harmless and well worth trying.

Formula for "Liverish" Migraine

Some authorities maintain that liver trouble is one of the most common among the many different causes of migraine headache. Normally the bile that forms in the cells of the liver is thin and clear and flows freely through the gall bladder ducts. The bladder empties periodically. But if the bile thickens (generally due to consumption of fatty and indigestible foodstuffs or some temporary congestion of the bile ducts), the flow is slow, and the gall bladder does not empty. This back-up of bile into the bloodstream is believed to be the cause of severe migraine headaches.

Once the thickened bile starts to flow, the nauseated, "liverish" migraine sufferer begins to vomit the greenish-yellow bile, sometimes every several hours both day and night, often for two or three days. When at long last the excess bile is completely eliminated, the headache is finally relieved. But so long as the backed-up bile is retained in the system, the nausea and blinding headache persist. Therefore, to get the bile flowing as soon as possible during a migraine attack and to keep it flowing more often, Chinese herbalists advise the sufferer to drink one or two glasses of plain hot water. Drinking the water usually starts an amount of the bile flowing which can then be eliminated through vomiting. The glasses of water are continued every hour or two as needed, until the excess bile is completely eliminated. This means of washing out the bile from the system shortens the duration of the attack and more quickly relieves the blinding migraine headaches.

Although the hot water treatment may bring more prompt relief during a spell of "liverish" migraine, it will not cure the condition. That is, it will not prevent future attacks from occurring. Therefore, the real aim is to heal the ailment and produce lasting results. Following are examples of Chinese herb formulas which have reputedly proved helpful in a number of cases of "liverish" migraine.

One-half ounce each of vervain, dandelion root, ginger root, marshmallow root, motherwort, wild carrot (*Daucus carota*), centaury (*Erythraea centaurium*), and fringe tree (*Chionanthus virginicus*) are mixed together and simmered in one quart of boiling water for fifteen minutes in a covered vessel. The decoction is strained, and one teacupful is taken three times a day before meals. This formula is taken for several weeks, or longer if necessary, because the effects are reputedly slow and gradual. It is said that the periods between the migraine attacks should lengthen, and the severity of the attacks should lessen.

A Notable Ingredient

Although each herb listed in the above formula is considered very valuable, the botanical known as fringe tree deserves special attention since the Chinese have reported good effects on "liverish" migraine from the employment of this one herb alone. It is used in the form of a fluid extract, 12 drops in a little warm water, three times a day after meals. No milk should be taken. The Chinese claim that milk is *yin* and works against the medicinal action of fringe tree.

The fluid extract of fringe tree combined with the fluid extract of an herb known as Greater Celandine (*Chelidonium majus*) is another remedy which has reportedly brought relief to sufferers of "liverish" migraine. Equal amounts of the two fluid extracts are mixed together, and one teaspoonful in a little warm water is taken three times daily after meals. (In some instances, this combination has also been known to dissolve gallstones, when the treatment is continued long enough.)

Another remedy, consisting of equal parts of the fluid extracts of fringe tree and poke root mixed together, is reputed to be a good liver alterative and therefore helpful in relieving conditions of "liverish" migraine headaches. One-half to one teaspoonful of the combined fluid extracts is taken in a small glass of warm water three times daily after meals.

Dietary Tips and Accessory Treatment for "Liverish" Migraine

In addition to the use of the herb remedies for "liverish" migraine, the Chinese advise sufferers to avoid eating or drinking anything cold. All foods or fluids should be warm or hot. It is also claimed that victims of this type of migraine headache are sensitive to external cold as well as internal cold. Therefore, the body should never be permitted to become chilled, especially in the upper abdomen and waist areas. In cold weather, extra warm clothing should be worn around the bodily areas mentioned, and any exposure to strong winds should be avoided at all times.

Fried foods and dairy products such as milk, cream, eggs, and cheese are to be omitted from the diet. If the person is troubled with irregularity, steps should be taken to keep the bowels open. This may be accomplished with the use of natural aids. (Refer to the chapter on bowel complaints.)

As a dietary supplement, one tablespoonful of lecithin granules obtained from soybeans (obtainable from health food stores) may be taken twice daily. (Lecithin reputedly has a beneficial effect on the liver and gall bladder.) The granules may be sprinkled over foods or added to fluids such as soups, coffee, or juices.

The amount of lecithin granules cited rarely if ever disagrees, but there are exceptions, and a few people find it too rich. In such cases, the amount is simply reduced or may be completely cut out.

WU-CHIA-P'I

English Name: Eleuthero
Botanical Name: *Eleutherococcus senticosus*

This tall shrub grows wild in various areas of the Far East and belongs to the same Araliaceae family as Panax ginseng. The flowers are violet or yellowish, and the leaves are similar in appearance to those of ginseng. Because its branches are spiked with thorns, people in olden times called the plant Touch-me-not and Devil's Bush, and these synonyms are still in use today. More modern names for the Eleutherococcus bush are simple Eleuthero (pronounced El-oo-ther-oh) and "Siberian Ginseng."

In China, eleuthero is employed as a tonic and as a remedy for a great number of disorders, including nervousness and stress. It is generally used in the form of a tincture or extract.

Russian Scientific Studies on Eleuthero

Soviet scientists have taken a great interest in Chinese herbs and have discovered that eleuthero, a member of the ginseng family, is not only native to various areas of China, but also grows wild and abundantly in southern regions of the Soviet Union. It is for this reason, and the fact that the plant has undergone years of scientific study by a battery of Russian researchers at the Far Eastern Center of the Siberian Division of the USSR Academy of Sciences, that the herb is called "Siberian Ginseng." Results of these tests have established that eleutherococcus possesses an incredibly wide range of therapeutic activity, thereby substantiating many of the claims made for the herb by the Chinese. For example, prepared as a fluid extract and used as a tonic, it restores loss of vigor and vitality, increases endurance, gives more mental alertness, and so on. As a remedy, it reduces elevated sugar content in mild and moderate cases of diabetes, normalizes low blood pressure and mild forms of high blood pressure, protects against stress, has a beneficial effect in functional nervous disorders, and much more.

In this chapter we will briefly consider some of the Russian studies on eleuthero in relation to nerve conditions and stress. For more thorough detailed coverage of the many Soviet scientific studies on the therapeutic effects of eleuthero, plus case histories, see the book *Eleuthero—Health Herb of Russia,* which is available at health food stores.

Anti-Stress Action of Eleuthero on Animals

Russian scientists have established that a preparation of eleuthero has a marked protective action against most types of stress. For example, lengthy series of experiments on animals involved stress factors such as increased muscle loads, swimming for long durations, exposure to extreme heat and cold, chemical intoxication, surgery, and confinement in a closed vessel. In all of these experiments it was found that where eleuthero extract was administered, an anti-stress action was produced. For instance, one group of rats was injected with a preparation of eleuthero, and a second group was not. One hour later, both groups were made to swim in water until absolute exhaustion (death). The group not receiving the plant extract all developed bloating of the adrenals; decreased adrenal ascorbic acid; and shriveling of the thymus, spleen, and lymph nodes. Among the rats that received eleuthero, these destructive changes were hindered. It was also noted that the endurance of the treated rats increased remarkably. In comparison to the first group, they were able to swim fifty-two minutes longer until total fatigue (death).

Studies on Anti-Stress Action of Eleuthero on Humans

Under strict Soviet scientific guide-lines, the anti-stress effect of eleuthero was studied on humans. After a long-term series of tests that took years, it was concluded that the plant extract increases human resistance to a wide variety of stress factors. The herb preparation helped people cope better under the ordinary stress and tension of modern everyday living; counteracted threats to typical stress-induced illnesses; produced a soothing and calming effect on people who had endured months of pressure and tension; eased the strain of worry and bottled up anxiety; relieved tensions of business and sports competitions; and delivered a protective effect against the stress of surgery, accidents, certain chemical toxins, radiation, and chronic illnesses.

In brief, Soviet scientists have firmly established that for people who find themselves in a trying situation or those who are engaged in any activity which taxes their endurance or stresses their body in other ways eleuthero extract can provide a protection that enables them to get through these periods with far less damage than they might otherwise incur.

Eleuthero Tested on Nervous Disorders

Probing further into the secrets of eleuthero, Soviet experts discovered that the plant extract had a pronounced therapeutic effect on functional nervous disorders, even in chronic patients who had been previously treated by a variety of different medications which had not helped.

Clinical studies with the plant extract were carried out on patients suffering from nervous exhaustion or nervous and emotional disturbances (not insanity). Their symptoms ranged from hair-trigger irritability to moodiness, lethargy, apprehension, menopausal "blues," anxiety, feelings of impending doom, fears of heart trouble or insanity, persistent insomnia, depression, loss of vigor, and chronic fatigue.

In most patients, the administration of eleuthero extract brought about an improvement in sleep, a restoration of energy and strength, a marked sense of well-being, and a renewed interest in life and work. The extract also displayed its normalizing effects in many areas. For example, while relieving symptoms of weakness, exhaustion, moodiness, and depression in patients suffering from these conditions, it produced a calm, restful, and well balanced effect on emotionally excited patients.

How Eleuthero Was Administered

The eleuthero treatment in these cases of nervous exhaustion and nervous and emotional disturbances lasted for four to five weeks. One dose of twenty to forty drops of the extract was taken three times a day. To achieve a stable therapeutic effect, Dr. Brekhman, a prominent member of the Soviet scientific team, says: "It is recommended to give two or three courses at one or two week intervals." He adds that: "The preparations from eleutherococcus are non-toxic and harmless even when administered recurringly over a long period of time."

Note: A "course" means one month or five weeks of daily doses of eleuthero extract. At the end of that time, the doses are discontinued for one or two weeks, and then another course of eleuthero is taken.

Eleuthero—Widely Used

Eleutherococcus senticosus extract is manufactured for use and widely available to the Russian public. In addition, a cold drink called "Bodrost" (cheerfulness) contains eleuthero and is very popular among the Russian people.

In one of the reports published by Soviet scientists in an International Congress, eleutherococcus was included in the list of therapeutic agents which can be of interest for space medicine (e.g. to help protect Russian cosmonauts against stress and to give them better endurance in space.)

Eleutherococcus senticosus extract is currently available in the United States and can be obtained from health food stores or herb companies.

MI-TIEH-HSIANG

English Name: Rosemary
Botanical Name: *Rosmarinus officinalis*

There are several varieties of rosemary, such as the silver and gold leaves under cultivation in gardens, but the variety known as *Rosmarinus officinalis,* a small shrub with pale blue flowers and fragrant evergreen leaves, is the kind used medicinally. Its botanical name comes from the Latin *ros,* dew, and *marinus,* of the sea, since the wild plant grows abundantly near the seashore. This herb was introduced into China from Rome many centuries ago.

Medicinal Uses

Rosemary contains a special camphor, a volatile oil, a bitter principle, and a resin. Prepared as a tea, it reputedly soothes the nerves and relieves nervous insomnia, mental fatigue, and simple or congestive headaches. One heaping teaspoonful of the cut leaves is placed in a cup, and boiling water is added. The infusion is covered with a saucer, allowed to stand for five minutes, and then strained. One cupful of the hot tea is sipped slowly three or four times a day between meals.

Spirits of Rosemary

Here is another method of using rosemary for the relief of simple or congestive headache. As soon as the headache begins, a small bottle of spirits of rosemary is held to the nose, and the fumes are inhaled. In addition, a few drops of the preparation is rubbed gently but thoroughly on the temples, on the forehead, on the veins of the neck, and behind the ears. This treatment reputedly gives prompt relief.

Combined Rosemary Tea Formulas

As a remedy for nervous sick headache, one-half teaspoonful each of rosemary, sage, and peppermint leaves is placed with the others in a cup which is filled with boiling water. The cup is covered with a saucer, and the tea is allowed to stand for five minutes and then strained. One cup of the hot tea is sipped slowly every hour or two until relief is obtained.

In a few instances migraine headache sufferers have reported relief with the use of a formula consisting of one ounce each of rosemary, scullcap, vervain, and wood betony *(Betonica officinalis).* The herbs are thoroughly mixed together, and one ounce of the mixture is placed in one pint of cold water and brought to a boil. The container is covered, and the tea is simmered for two minutes and then allowed to stand until cold. The tea is then strained, reheated, and taken warm—one teacupful three times a day between meals and once before bedtime. The tea is used daily until relief is felt.

One woman who suffered periodic bouts of migraine for six years reported permanent relief after several weeks' use of the above herbal formula.

AI-HAO

English Name: Mugwort
Botanical Name: *Artemisia vulgaris*

This plant is the common mugwort, known in China as *Ai-hao* or simply *Ai.* It is found in most parts of China. In Chinese commerce it is sold principally in three forms—*Ai-yeh,* the dried leaves; *Ai-t'iao,* the dried twigs tied in bundles; and *Ai-jung,* which is made by taking the best dried leaves and grinding them in a stone mortar with water, removing the coarsest particles and refuse, then drying and powdering what remains.

An Ancient Healing Art

Solely as an item of interest, it may be noted that besides acupuncture, the Chinese use "moxibustion," which differs only in its method of application—heat produced by burning mugwort is used instead of a needle. The *Ai-jung* (mugwort powder) is made into cones called moxas and applied to acupuncture points under the strict supervision of a Chinese practitioner. In the ancient Chinese text, the *Nei Ching,* we find: "For all ailments in which acupuncture is forbidden, moxas must be used. The mugwort from which they are made has the power of extracting the Yang energy from the Yin."

The base of the mugwort cone is placed on the skin, and the tip of the cone is ignited. It does not burn with a flame, but smolders somewhat like incense. To protect the skin from overheating and scarring, a thin slice of ginger or garlic is placed between the skin and moxa cone.

Moxibustion treatment must never be attempted by a layman. It is a refined and complex technique which requires great skill and years of training. Essentially, success depends on the Chinese practitioner applying exactly the right amount of heat to the exact points on the body, but other factors are also considered—such as the number of moxa cones used and the number of treatments required.

Mugwort Venerated as a Charm

According to an ancient Chinese almanac, people gathered mugwort at the time of the Dragon Festival (the fifth day of the fifth moon) and hung the herb up in the home or on the front door or door posts as a charm against evil influences. Sometimes this was also done either with a Taoist charm, in which case it was called *Ai-fu* and hung in the principal rooms of the house, or with the herb *Acorus calamus,* which was formed in the shape of a sword and placed over the door, while a stalk of mugwort was hung on each door post.

That mugwort was an effective charm in one instance is attested to by the fact that the famous Chinese rebel, Huang Ch'ao ordered his soldiers to spare the lives of any family or individual in whose home mugwort could be found!

Mugwort Tea in Chinese Medicine

Medicinally, mugwort tea is cited as a nervine, tonic, stimulant, diaphoretic, and emmenagogue. As a nervine, the tea is prepared in a covered vessel. One pint of boiling water is poured over one heaping tablespoon of the dried leaves. The tea is allowed to stand for fifteen minutes and then strained. It is best taken in small doses—one warm teacupful in the morning and one in the evening or one tablespoonful three or four times a day. (Mugwort has a very bitter taste and may be sweetened with a little honey.)

The Chinese maintain that mugwort tea is often helpful in relieving conditions of sleep-walking. This particular beneficial effect has also been commented upon by various Western herbalists. For example, C.F. Lyle writes: "The connection between the brain and the spinal cord is so intimate that herbs which affect the spine are likely to have some action on the brain. Mugwort, for instance, stimulates the spinal cord and relieves congestion in the brain. Sleep-walking is often combatted by mugwort. It is a good brain tonic."

Mugwort Fomentations

Fomentations of mugwort reputedly bring relief in torticollis (neuritis of the neck muscles), a condition symptomized by a spasm or contraction of the muscles on one side of the neck which causes the head to be tilted. One quart of boiling water is poured over one ounce of mugwort, the container is covered, and the infusion is allowed to stand for fifteen minutes and then strained. A small towel, dressing, or similar material is dipped into the tea, quickly wrung out and applied to the area, and covered with a dry towel. When the dressing completely dries, the same procedure is repeated three or four times. This routine is followed once daily and must be continued for lasting results.

SUMMARY

1. Centuries of Chinese experience have shown that specific herbal aids for coping with jittery nerves, tension, insomnia, and nagging headache pains are effective, harmless, and non-habit forming.
2. The pains of certain types of neuritis have often yielded to the use of herbs in various forms such as teas, fomentations, or poultices.
3. Due to the diversity of causes of the ailments covered in this chapter, a select herb remedy may help one person but not another. By choosing one remedy at a time and giving it a sufficient trial, you may be able to find the formula most suitable to your own personal needs.
4. In addition to using herbs, faulty dietary habits must be changed. Junk foods are to be replaced with wholesome, well-balanced meals. The Chinese also advise that insomniacs cut down on salt in their diets.
5. Because food must have time to digest, you should never retire immediately after eating a meal. This practice has been known to cause nightmares and restlessness. Sufficient sleep is necessary so that energy lost during the day may be restored to exhausted bodies.
6. According to Chinese herbalists, liver trouble is one of the most common causes of migraine headache. In addition to the use of herbs, the Chinese advise the sufferer of "liverish" migraine to avoid eating or drinking anything cold. Dairy products such as milk, cheese, eggs, and cream, as well as fried foods, are also to be omitted from the diet. If the sufferer is troubled with constipation, steps should be taken to restore and insure regularity by means of natural aids.

13

PLANT REMEDIES FOR CIRCULATORY DISORDERS

A Word about Hypertension

In medical terms, high blood pressure is known as *hypertension.* Blood pressure means the force of the blood against the walls of the arteries. When the pressure is abnormally high, it naturally causes abnormal wear and tear on the blood vessels. In severe cases, the pressure can cause the strained capillaries (tiny blood vessels) to rupture, which may result in a heart attack or stroke (cerebral hemorrhage). Stroke is the third leading cause of death in the United States. The brain is believed to be particularly susceptible to hemorrhage because it is enclosed in the skull and cannot expand when the blood pressure increases.

Kidney diseases, particularly inflammation, can cause hypertension, however only a very small percentage of the cases of high blood pressure are accounted for by kidney disease. More common is that type of high blood pressure known as "essential hypertension." This type is presumed to exist without any well-defined cause being known.

The usual symptoms of high blood pressure are dizziness, headaches, and noises or ringing in the ears. Along with any remedy used for hypertension, the following regime is generally recommended: sufficient rest; regular exercise; abstinence from tobacco, coffee, and alcoholic beverages; a low-salt diet; minimization or, if possible, avoidance of stress provoking situations; and control of the cholesterol count by correct diet or other means.

A Word about Hypotension

Low blood pressure is medically called *hypotension*. In this condition the push or force of blood against the vessel walls decreases, and the cells fail to receive an adequate supply of nutrients carried by the blood. Fatigue, sensitivity to cold and heat, rapid pulse beat on exertion, and lack of endurance are the usual symptoms of low blood pressure. A person with this condition requires more sleep than a healthy individual and generally finds himself more tired when he awakens in the morning than when he went to bed.

CHINESE HERB REMEDIES FOR CIRCULATORY DISORDERS

WU-CHIA-P'I

English Name: Eleuthero; "Siberian Ginseng"
Botanical Name: *Eleutherococcus senticosus*

Prepared as an extract, this member of the ginseng family is used as a natural remedy for normalizing the blood pressure, raising the pressure if it is too low and reducing it in mild or moderate conditions of high blood pressure. Yet this action does not interfere with normal blood pressure. Therefore, the extract may be used for other purposes—e.g., those cited in the chapter on nerve tension and stress—without concern that it will disturb normal blood pressure.

Although eleuthero extract has proved effective in many instances in relieving mild or moderate forms of hypertension, it is cited as especially effective (a specific) for conditions of low blood pressure.

Scientific Studies of Eleuthero on Blood Pressure

Results of carefully controlled studies by Soviet scientists have established that eleuthero extract does indeed have a normalizing effect on blood pressure. Dr. Brekhman writes: "It is known that eleutherococcus is one of the best remedies for curing hypotension [low blood pressure] but at the same time it reduces the elevated blood pressure in many hypertensive [high blood pressure] patients, or, in other words, displays its normalizing, adaptogenic action."[1] He points out that in conditions of high blood pressure the reduction is gradual and moderate, except in severe forms of high blood pressure, which do not respond to the eleuthero extract.

How Eleuthero Extract Is Used

Dr. Brekhman recommends from twenty to forty drops of the extract in a little water to be taken before meals two or three times a day, to make the total daily dose of eighty drops. The course of treatment lasts for twenty-five to thirty days. If necessary the course may be repeated again at one or two week intervals. In other words, when one course has been completed the treatment is discontinued for one or two weeks, after which another course of twenty-five to thirty days treatment is taken.

HU-TS'UNG

English Name: Onion
Botanical Name: *Allium cepa*

There are several varieties of onions native to China, but the common onion which is largely cultivated in the Southern regions of the land is believed to be of foreign origin. It is called *Hu-ts'ung* and *Hui-hui-ts'ung*—the latter term meaning "Mohammedan onion," indicating its derivation from the West.

In China the onion is a favorite article of the diet. It is eaten with rice, millet, or bread, together with green vegetables.

Medicinal Uses

The onion belongs to the same botanical family as garlic and leeks and has been used for centuries for treating a host of different ailments ranging from circulatory disorders to the common cold. Because of its incredibly wide range of usage, onions are employed in a variety of forms—for example, freshly extracted onion juice; onions eaten raw, boiled, roasted, fried, or baked; chopped or grated onions applied as compresses or prepared as hot poultices; teas made with onions; finely grated onions mixed with honey or prepared as syrups; and so on.

---

[1]Lucas, R., *Eleuthero—Health Herb of Russia* (Spokane, Washington: R & M Books, 1972), pp. 29-30.

In this chapter we will restrict our attention to the Chinese usage of onions in relation to circulatory disorders. The Chinese maintain that onions relieve high blood pressure; help eliminate fluid in the cardiac and pleural sacs; and, when eaten boiled or fried, will help prevent or dissolve dangerous blood clots.

Modern Medical Report on Onions

The Western medical profession is taking considerable interest in the therapeutic possibilities of onions for treating high blood pressure and other problems of the circulatory system. For example, a team of British doctors has demonstrated with tests on humans that boiled or fried onions can help reduce the possibility of heart attacks by raising the blood's ability to prevent or dissolve deadly clots. This information was reported in the following article which appeared in the *West London Observer:*

ONIONS AND THROMBOSIS

In France, horses who develop clots in the legs are treated with garlic and onions. A chance statement to this effect by a human patient led four Newcastle doctors to investigate the possible effect of onions on blood clotting.

The essential element in the formation of a clot is the change of substance called fibrinogen in the blood to insoluble fibrin, which forms a fine mesh; the "scaffolding" of the clot.

The blood of a healthy person has a measurable ability to "dissolve" this fibrin—a fibrinolytic activity, as doctors call it—and it has been known for some time that a fatty meal reduces this activity.

Would onions stop this reduction or even reverse it, and so make the formation of a clot unlikely? This is the question the four doctors tried to answer.

They gave a fatty breakfast to each of twenty-two patients, and confirmed that two or three hours later the fibrinolytic activity of their blood certainly was reduced.

On a separate occasion they gave the same patients the same fatty breakfast, accompanied by two ounces of onions, fried for some of the patients, boiled for others.

Two or three hours later the fibrinolytic activity of their blood was found to be markedly increased; and the odds against the change being a chance finding were found to be less than 1 in 1,000. Research is now proceeding to discover which substance in onions could be responsible for this dramatic effect.

Is it of any importance?—Well, everyone knows that man, and particularly modern man, is plagued by clotting disease—thrombosis of leg veins, for instance, and more important, of coronary arteries.

Anything that will increase the blood's fibrinolytic activity might be very important in the treatment or prevention of these conditions; and all the known drugs that have fibrinolytic activity have some undesirable characteristic. Onions might provide the answer.

In the meantime, one might speculate on why onions, fried or in a stuffing, are the traditional accompaniment to such fatty foodstuffs as steak and pork and goose, and why they are almost invariably cooked in fat. Has man's instinct been a few centuries ahead of his reason?

Whatever the truth may turn out to be, onion and garlic addicts need apologize much less in future, while at medical banquets the leek, that close relative of the onion, will doubtless be de rigueur, acceptable at once to both the social and the professional conscience of the diners.

Note: Pharmaceutical firms are now busy searching for the basic ingredient in onions that may lead to the development of a cheap, non-harmful medication.

SANG

English Name: Mulberry Tree
Botanical Name: *Morus alba*

The cultivation of the mulberry tree in China dates from antiquity. According to ancient tradition, Si-ling, the empress of Huangti (B.C. 2967), taught the people how to use mulberry leaves for rearing silk worms. (Silk worms feed upon mulberry leaves.)

Several varieties of the tree are found in all parts of China. The *fruits* of the common mulberry *(Morus alba)* are known as *Shen.* When fully ripened they are called *Hsun* or *T'an.* In commerce they are sold under the name *Sang-shen-tzu* and made into a jam called *Sang-shen-kao,* in which form the fruits are preserved for medicinal purposes.

Therapeutic Uses

The juice of the ripe berries, diluted with water and used in considerable quantities, is reputed to improve the circulation and to have a tonic effect on the heart. It is also said to produce diuresis and

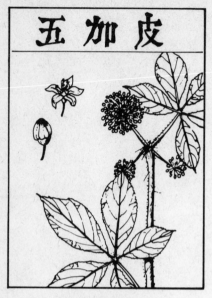

WU-CHIA-P'I
(Eleutherococcus)

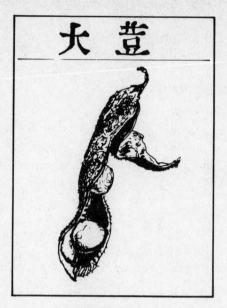

TA-TOU
(Soy Bean)

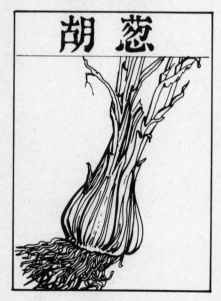

HU-TS'UNG
(Onion)

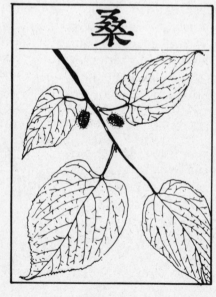

SANG
(Mulberry)

therefore to be helpful in some instances for relieving conditions of cardiac dropsy.

A Scientific Study

According to a medical report, eighteen heart patients were treated by mulberry therapy, and all but two showed marked improvement. Pain and shortness of breath were reduced, and in some cases swelling of the ankles vanished.

SUAN

English Name: Garlic
Botanical Name: *Allium sativum*

In China garlic has a long-standing reputation as a near specific for forms of hypertension symptomized by dizziness, noises or ringing in the ears, and difficulty in concentrating, and especially for that form accompanying arteriosclerosis with anxiety feelings. Over the centuries, the learned Chinese herbalists, along with many of the common people and royalty, all testified that garlic was a normalizer of high blood pressure. It is said that an emperor of China cured himself of hypertension solely with the use of garlic.

Note: High blood pressure caused by kidney disease does not respond to garlic treatment.

How Garlic Is Used

For relieving high blood pressure, fresh garlic may be chopped and added liberally to foods or garlic perles may be used. The perles contain garlic oil. They provide the full benefit of garlic nutrients but leave no odor on your breath since they do not dissolve until they have reached the lower digestive tract.

Generally, one to three garlic perles are swallowed with a small amount of water three times daily. When the blood pressure has been normalized, the amount of garlic is reduced to maintenance dosages.

Scientific Evidence

Modern medical evidence for garlic as a remedy in cases of high blood pressure are too numerous to cite, but a few examples may be given as follows:

• French scientist Poullard reported that garlic reduces high blood pressure.

• From lengthy experiments on both humans and animals, Loeper and De Bray found that garlic causes a decided drop in blood pressure in cases of hypertension.

• Consistant reduction in blood pressure in eighty cases of hypertension treated with garlic was reported by Ortner in Germany.

• Schlesinger cited a drop in pressure after fifteen days' treatment with garlic.

• De Seze and Gaulien also reported that garlic was effective in relieving high blood pressure.

• Kristine Nolfi, M.D., of Denmark, wrote that garlic "lowers too high blood pressure and raises one which is too low."[2] [This action reputedly does not interfere with normal blood pressure.]

• In a European journal, *Praxis,* Dr. F.G. Piotrowski, a member of the faculty of medicine at the University of Geneva, wrote an article in which he related his experiences with the use of garlic in treating about 100 hypertensive patients. Patients with renal hypertension (high blood pressure caused by malfunction or disease of the kidneys) were not included in the test.

Dr. Piotrowski reported that in 40% of the cases he obtained a drop of at least two centimeters in blood pressure. Subjective symptoms such as headaches, dizziness, angina-like pains, back pains, and difficulty in concentrating began to disappear within three to five days after administration of garlic oil was begun. He explained that in treating his patients he started by administering fairly large doses, which were gradually diminished over a period of three weeks. He then continued with smaller doses for the balance of the treatment. The patients were all allowed to go about their daily work, so bed rest or inactivity did not have a chance to influence the results. They claimed that they could think more clearly and perform their jobs better.

Dr. Piotrowski also mentioned that the expected drop of two centimeters in blood pressure usually takes place after about a week of garlic treatment. He concluded his article by recommending that many more doctors include garlic therapy in treating hypertensive patients.

---

[2]*My Experiences with Living Food,* p. 11.

TA-TOU

English Name: Soybeans
Botanical Name: *Glycine hispidia*

The soybean has an ancient history. It was cultivated in China more than four thousand years ago and was considered one of the five sacred grains along with rice, barley, wheat, and millet. The renowned Taoist doctor Szu-miao, who lived at the beginning of the Tang period and who was given the honored title of "King of Medicaments," was the first to note the various types of soybeans, such as Ta-tou and Wu-tou.

In China, the soybean has been nicknamed "China Cow" because it produces so much protein that for generations it has been used in many parts of the land as a substitute for milk. The soybean is also employed in many Chinese food preparations such as soy flour and soy relish, but the three that are of almost universal use in Oriental cookery are soybean oil, soy sauce, and soybean curd.

Soybeans in the United States

The first soybeans were brought to the United States in 1804 by a Yankee clipper ship returning from China. A few people sowed the seeds and perpetuated the plant, but there wasn't much interest in the plant. It was not until well over a century later, during World War II, that the American people began to realize the full potential of the valuable plant, and farmers throughout the country began to grow the bean in increasing numbers.

Today, many hundreds of millions of bushels of soybeans are grown yearly in the U.S. This remarkable legume is the only member of the plant kingdom which gives complete protein comparable to all forms of animal meats. Soybeans contain 11 times as much protein as milk, twice as much protein as meat or fish, and one and one-half times as much protein as cheese.

Other Valuable Nutrients

Along with an abundance of protein, soybeans also contain vitamins A, E, K, and some of the B factors. Other nutrients found in the beans include potassium, iron, phosphorus, calcium, and amino acids. In addition, soybeans are rich in unsaturated fatty acids of which the most important is *lecithin*.

Lecithin for Coping with Cholesterol

Lecithin is composed of bland, water-soluble granules refined from soybeans and is available from health food stores and various herb firms. Many Chinese-American herbalists recommend soybean lecithin as a dietary supplement, claiming that it helps regulate the metabolism, reduces cholesterol, and supplies nutriment to the brain, nerves, and glandular and sexual system.

Cholesterol is a major ingredient of plaque, a build-up of fatty particles that frequently become deposited within the arteries. When the arteries become clogged, blood circulation to all parts of the body, especially to the brain, is reduced. This shortage of blood to the brain can cause mental confusion, forgetfulness, and high blood pressure. Deposits of fatty particles also cause the heart to work harder in order to pump the blood through the clogged passage ways. Here is where many heart and coronary troubles begin, if the heart is forced to undertake more work than it is able to do.

Cholesterol build-up can also bring about complications such as nervousness, gallstones, eczema, psoriasis, a certain type of arthritis, and atherosclerosis (hardening of the arteries).

How Lecithin Is Used

As dietary supplements, generally one tablespoonful of granular soybean lecithin is taken twice daily and one or two tablespoonfuls of soybean oil are taken daily. The granules may be used in any number of ways, e.g., stirred in juices, sprinkled over cereals, and added to meat or vegetable dishes. The oil may be used over salads and as cooking oil.

Proper diet is also stressed. Animal fats should be avoided because they have a high prevalence of cholesterol. Foods fried in deep fat or prepared with saturated fats should be greatly reduced or completely cut out. The same applies to pies, cakes, and other pastries that are prepared with hydrogenated shortening or synthetic fats. The more hydrogenated or saturated ·fats you consume, the more lecithin you need to handle them.

The time required for relieving or preventing cholesterol deposits by taking soybean lecithin varies with each person.

Note: Lecithin is also available in capsules and in liquid form.

Scientific Evaluation and Reported Uses

Many of the Chinese claims for the therapeutic value of lecithin is supported by modern medicine findings:

• In an article published some years ago in the *Journal of the Mt. Sinai Hospital,* David Adlersberg, M.D. and Harry Sobotka, Ph.D. reported on five cases of high cholesterol in which a "striking decrease in serum cholesterol level was achieved by addition of commercial lecithin to the diet." One woman, age 41, had a cholesterol count of 620. She began taking 12 grams (two table-spoonfuls) of soybean lecithin daily, and in two months her count was down to 420. After another month, her count was down to 300. Another woman, 38 years of age, was troubled with multiple health problems, including high cholesterol in her blood and fatty deposits in her skin. Her extremely high cholesterol count of 1370 was sharply reduced to 445 when she took 15 grams of lecithin a day for a period of three months. The cholesterol count of a 35 year old man dropped from 440 to 260 while he was taking two tablespoonfuls of lecithin daily for two months.

Another case was that of a 55-year-old woman who was diabetic and very obese. Her cholesterol count was 360. Six weeks later, after she took a little more than two tablespoons of lecithin every day, her count had dropped to 235. To see what would happen, the doctors took her off the lecithin and found that her cholesterol count rapidly rose again.

• The staff of the *British Medical Journal* recommends soybean oil for treating an excess of cholesterol in the blood, adding that the oil may also help in preventing blood clots and heart attacks.

• After many years of careful analyses and evaluation, Dr. Lester M. Morrison says that he is "certain that lecithin is one of our most powerful weapons against disease." He adds that it "is an especially valuable bulwark against development of 'hardening of the arteries' and all the complications of heart, brain, and kidney that follow." He also feels that soya oil is "the most healthful of all food oils."

Dr. Morrison cited many cases in which the cholesterol count was reduced with the use of lecithin. To mention one example, he reported that 12 out of 15 patients experienced an average reduction of serum cholesterol of 156 milligrams after three months of taking soybean lecithin supplements daily. He points out that a low-fat diet alone had failed to lower the cholesterol level in these patients.

Dr. Morrison also mentions that two of these patients had a history of angina pains, but after they took lecithin for three months "the symptoms of angina disappeared . . . "

The intitial amount of 36 grams (6 tablespoons) of lecithin administered by Dr. Morrison is relatively high. However, he reported that follow-up work indicated that a maintenance dose of one or two tablespoons of lecithin daily was effective in sustaining normal cholesterol levels. (Normal cholesterol levels are said to range from 200 to 250 milligrams.)[3]

• A 60-year-old man with dangerously high blood pressure and severe nose bleeds spent a month in the hospital. When he returned home, his doctors were not very optimistic about his condition. He began taking a tablespoon of lecithin daily for three months, and his blood pressure dropped over one hundred points.

• In an article published in the *American Laboratory* (July, 1973), Jacobus Rinse, Ph.D., a chemist, wrote that back in 1951 he suffered severe angina attacks. His physician told him he had ten years to live, providing he carefully avoided all types of strenuous exercise. Drawing on his knowledge of chemistry, Dr. Rinse theorized that taking soybean lecithin would help keep the cholesterol liquified in his system. He began a dietary program of using supplements, which included one tablespoon of soybean lecithin granules and a tablespoon each of raw wheat germ, bone meal, brewer's yeast, and soybean or safflower oil. He used this mixture in cereals and occasionally in yogurt.

He reported that for years, since he began taking these dietary supplements, he has never been troubled with angina. He also cited the experiences of many friends and acquaintances with circulatory problems who said they were benefitted by a nutritional program featuring lecithin.

Multiple Benefits

Numerous reports also back up the Chinese claim that there are many other benefits that can be traced to the addition of soybean lecithin in the diet. Following are some examples.

• A nurse said that external applications of liquid lecithin successfully cleared up her infant's persistent diaper rash. Another

---

[3]*The Low Fat Way to Health and Longer Life* (Englewood Cliffs, N.J.: Prentice-Hall, Inc., 1958).

nurse who heard about it thought that liquid lecithin might possibly heal bedsores in hospital patients. To try out the therapy, she selected a gentleman patient (at the hospital where she worked) who was weak and frail and had two bedsores on the lower spine.

The nurse obtained permission of the patient's doctor to apply external applications of liquid lecithin to the bedsores. Several other nurses cooperated, and on each shift the bedsores were first cleansed with hydrogen peroxide, then coated with liquid lecithin and bandaged with a non-stick dressing. The dressing was changed at least three times during a twenty-four hour period. Care was also taken to keep the patient off the bedsore area by correct positioning of his body.

The nurse reports that they were all greatly surprised to find that definite improvement was noticeable within two to three days. She adds that the patient is still in the hospital and very ill, but the bedsores seem to be healing nicely. Since hospital pharmacies do not stock lecithin, she explains, she purchased it at a local health food store.

• Dr. Dietrick of El Paso, Texas reported that he has treated many diabetic patients successfully with lecithin. He found that after a few weeks of lecithin the insulin requirement gradually decreased, and eventually the patients were able to return to a normal diet. Dr. Dietrick says that the cure was accomplished with six tablespoonfuls of lecithin and one hundred milligrams of vitamin E daily. He adds: "It would seem quite possible that the cells of the pancreas which secrete insulin may have become starved for lecithin due to an insufficiency in the diet, and that for this reason they had reduced their manufacture of insulin. When sufficient lecithin is again supplied, it is quite conceivable that those cells might resume their normal secretion of insulin . . . "

• Mr. A.M.C. wrote:

"From October to December, 1958, my vision was so bad that I could not read newsprint. I saw my eye doctor, who said he could not do anything for it. I asked what caused it, and he said it was caused by bad circulation.

"Remembering an article I had read about lecithin, I began to take raw liquid lecithin, one teaspoon three times daily. Three weeks later my vision was restored to normal. I told my doctor about it and he said, 'Oh, yes, you have gotten your bloodstream cleared out.'"

• One man reported that hearing in his right ear had been impaired for many years and that he also frequently experienced a ringing sound. He said he was aware of the value of lecithin in cleaning the blood stream of cholesterol plaques and fatty particles, so he decided to try it and took a large amount of lecithin daily with his meals. He says: "Much to my surprise the ringing in my ears has stopped and there has been an improvement in my hearing. I don't know which of the elements of the lecithin has caused the improvement; I don't know how far the improvement may go. But I'm going to continue my lecithin program since its quite pleasant to not have that ringing in the ears."

• Success in treating psoriasis with soybean lecithin was reported by Drs. Paul Gross and Beatrice Kesten of the Department of Dermatology at the Columbia-Presbyterian Medical Center. The doctors placed 235 patients on lecithin and a low-fat diet. Because of the restricted diet, the medics considered it important to administer vitamin supplements such as A, D, and the B vitamins, but were certain that lecithin was the agent responsible for the therapeutic effects on the condition of psoriasis.

Of the 235 patients, 155 were considered adequately treated, and the rest either refused to cooperate or abandoned the program before definite conclusions could be reached. Of those who followed the regime, only thirty-seven experienced no improvement. Twenty-three became well and remained well after one year of treatment and three years of observation. Twenty-nine were highly pleased that their psoriasis was being controlled. The remaining sixty-six subjects showed some improvement, but required special ointments in addition to the lecithin.

• Other medical experimentations have credited lecithin for controlling psoriasis. In an article written by Dr. Herman Goodman, a leading dermatologist, he described a new medicine, "one of a group of lipids—fatlike chemicals—which include lecithin and vitamin A," which proved successful on a small number of psoriasis patients.

• In her book, *Let's Eat Right To Keep Fit,* Adele Davis wrote: "Even the stubborn eczema-like condition known as psoriasis usually disappears rapidly when salad oils and lecithin are added to the diet."[4]

• Dr. Edward Hewitt reported that he has observed great improvement and complete cures in several cases of mental illness

---

[4]*Let's Eat Right to Keep Fit* (New York: Harcourt, Brace & World, Inc., 1954), p. 38.

when sufficient lecithin was added to the diet. He also maintains that many cases of arthritis are due to cholesterol deposits, and if arthritis is of this type lecithin added to the diet will effect a cure.

• According to Dr. R.K. Tompkins and his colleagues, all of Ohio State University College of Medicine, gallstones can be prevented when adequate lecithin is included in the diet. At an annual meeting of the Federation of American Societies for Experimental Biology, these investigators reported that "Over 90% of human gallstones are composed chiefly of cholesterol. The maintenance of cholesterol in solution in bile is the key to prevention of gallstone formation. Several investigations in recent years have suggested that a class of compounds called phospholipids are necessary for preventing cholesterol precipitation from bile. Our study indicates that human bile can be made richer in these phospholipids by feeding a commercial preparation of lecithin (obtained from soybeans), the principal phospholipid of bile. This increase in phospholipid content of human bile appears to enhance the ability of the bile to hold cholesterol in solution."

• In addition to lowering the cholesterol content of the blood and being a potent agent against development of hardening of the arteries and all the complications that follow, according to Dr. Lester Morrison, "Lecithin has other remarkable therapeutic qualities as well. One that we are just beginning to explore is its ability to increase the gamma globulin content of the blood proteins. These gamma globulins are known to be associated with nature's protective force against the attacks of various infections in the body.

"In the bloodstream of patients who used lecithin as recommended, we found evidence of increased immunity against virus infections. This is of special interest, since scientists have reported finding this lecithin-induced immunity against pneumonia."

SUMMARY

1. When prepared as an extract, the plant known as Eleutherococcus reportedly normalizes the blood pressure, raising the pressure if it is too low and reducing it in mild or moderate cases of high blood pressure. Yet this action does not interfere in any way with normal blood pressure.
2. In conditions of hypertension the following regime is generally recommended: Adequate rest; regular exercise; abstinence from

tobacco, coffee, and alcoholic beverages; a low-salt diet; minimization or avoidance of stress provoking situations; and keeping the cholesterol count normal by correct diet or other means.

3. The Chinese maintain that the humble onion is helpful for relieving various types of circulatory disorders. It is reputed to be of special value as an aid for preventing or dissolving dangerous blood clots.

4. Garlic is considered a near specific remedy for high blood pressure, but is not effective in cases where hypertension is caused by kidney disease.

5. The diluted juice of ripe mulberries is said to improve the circulation and to produce a tonic effect upon the heart.

6. Cholesterol consists of fatty particles that frequently lump together and become deposited within the walls of the arteries.

7. Cholesterol build-up can cause complications such as nervousness, gallstones, eczema, psoriasis, high blood pressure, strokes, a certain type of arthritis, and various heart and coronary ailments such as hardening of the arteries.

8. Soybean lecithin, when added to the diet, acts as an emulsifying agent for cholesterol. When cholesterol tends to lump together, lecithin breaks it up into tiny particles, enabling it to circulate through the body and preventing it from solidifying or congealing into large lumps and clinging to the sides of the arteries.

9. In addition to lowering excessive cholesterol, soybean lecithin supplements provide many other remarkable health benefits.

LIST OF HERB DEALERS

The list of herb dealers below is given solely for the convenience of the reader for purchasing the herbs and herbal products described in this book. The dealers are not connected in any way with the author or publishers of this book. You may write for their catalogs or price lists since they also deal in mail orders.

Kwan Yin Chinese Herb Co.
P.O. Box 7617
Spokane, Wa. 99208

Golden Gate Herb Research, Inc.
140 Market Street
San Rafael, Ca. 94901

Haussmann's Pharmacy
534-536 W. Girard Ave.
Philadelphia, Pa. 19123

Indiana Botanic Gardens
P.O. Box 5
Hammond, Indiana 46325
(Herbalist Almanac 50¢)

K.D. Distributor, Ltd.
1038 South Grand Ave.
Los Angeles, Ca. 90015

Nature's Herb Company
281 Ellis Street
San Francisco, Ca. 94102
(Catalog 20¢)

Pacific Trends, Inc.
6414 Variel Ave.
Woodland Hills, Ca. 91364

Penn Herb Company
603 North 2nd Street
Philadelphia, Pa. 19123

In Canada
Albi Imports Ltd.
207 W. Hastings, # 915
Vancouver, B.C., Canada

Botanica
P.O. Box 88, Sta. "N"
Montreal, Quebec, Canada

Ginseng The Magick Roote Co.
1461 Crescent St.
Montreal, Quebec, Canada

Nu-Life Nutrition Ltd.
871 Beatty Street
Vancouver, B.C., Canada

Index

Garlic (Suan):
   bowel complaints, 194-198
   colds-coughs-asthma-bronchitis, 59-61
   hypertension, 223-224
   menstrual cramps, 169
   nasal congestion, 61
   protective power, 61-62
   supportive evidence, 64-65
   tonsillitis, 61
   tuberculosis, 62-64
   vaginal infection, 169-170
   valuable remedy, 59
Gastric ulcer:
   description, 27
   magaimo (Chinese yam), 16
General Compendium of Remedies, 19
Ginger (Chiang):
   stomach disorders, 28-29
   suppressed or retarded menstruation, 168
Ginko tree (Yin-hsing), 42-45
Ginseng (Jenshen):
   celebrities laud, 77-78
   female health, 168-169
   forms, 81-82
   growing habits, 73
   longevity, 79
   men's ailments, 143-145
   modern times, 76
   plaudits, 71-73
   precious, 73
   scientific evaluation, 78-79
   several varieties, 79-81
   stomach disorders, 32
   synonyms, 75-76
   tips on, 82
   United States, 76-77
Ginseng Complex, Korean, 87-88
Ginseng Roots Compound, Chinese Processed, 88-92
Golden Age, 94, 95
Gold thread (Huang-lien), 29-30, 66
Gout:
   celery, 109-111
   Chinese Instant Fo-Ti-Tieng Roots Tea,
   106-108
   foods to avoid, 104
   Queen of the Meadow, 111
   term, 103
Gum benzoin (An-hsi-hsiang), 56-57
Gums:
   denture irritated, 66
   loose, spongy, 68
   sore, 66
   ulcers, or bleeding, 67, 68

H

Hartwell, Jonathan, 69
Harvey, 18
Hay fever, 50
Headache, 201, 203, 206-209, 212-214
Hearing, 230
Heartburn, 33
Hemorrhoids, (piles), 174-176, 184-185,
   193-194
Hoarseness, 58, 59
Honey, 83, 85
Hops, (Lu-ts' ao):
   headaches, nervousness, insomnia, 202-206
   neuralgia, sciatica, rheumatism, lumbago,
   112
Huang Ti, 17
Hydrocele, 146
Hypertension, 217-218, 220, 223, 226, 228
Hypotension, 218

I

Impotence, 143
Incontinence, 118, 119, 122, 129
Indigestion (*see* Stomach disorders)
Influenza, 56
Insomnia, 201, 203, 211
Irritability, 203

J

Jacobson, enzymes in alfalfa, 40
Jin Sam Jung, 83-87
Juniper berries (Kuei), 119-122

K

Kidney and bladder stones, 116-117, 122,
   123, 125, 131, 134, 137
Kingto Nin Jiom, 47
Knotgrass (Pien-hsu), 45, 68, 122-123
Korean Ginseng Complex, 87-88

L

Laryngitis, 57, 58, 64
Laxative habit, 177
Layman, P. de B., 96-97
Lecithin, 226-231
Leucorrhea, 165-166, 169
Li Chung Yun, 94-96
Licorice root (Kan-ts' ao), 58
Ling Shu, 17
Li Shih Chen, 19, 20